# The Breaking of the Surgeons

Neil Hyman, M.D.

# Dedication

I dedicate this book to Naomi, EJ and Seth -- how lucky can one guy get?

# Table of Contents

Preface ............................................................................... 1

Chapter 1: The Way We Were .................................................. 9

Chapter 2: The Fantasy Football League .................................... 19

Chapter 3: On Activity, Achievement and the Clipboard Nurses ........... 41

Chapter 4: Melvin and the Tostitos ........................................... 65

Chapter 5: Infinite and Free .................................................... 80

Chapter 6: Soap and Great Service ........................................... 94

Chapter 7: Don't Say Yes ...................................................... 107

Chapter 8: Burnout .............................................................. 123

Chapter 9: JOMO ................................................................ 139

Chapter 10: Academic Medical Centers ..................................... 160

Chapter 11: Quality ............................................................. 174

Chapter 12: The Data Dump .................................................. 189

Chapter 13: DEI ................................................................. 199

Chapter 14: Reflections ........................................................ 222

About the Author ................................................................ 229

THE BREAKING OF THE SURGEONS

# Preface

I retired in late 2023 after approximately 40 years as a surgeon, residency included. I have no need or desire to tell "war stories," fabricate or embellish heroic tales of achievement or discuss my career. Over the years, surgeons have written many excellent books describing the history of surgery, various aspects of surgical life or the remarkable achievements of luminaries in the field.

Rather, I have witnessed so many aspects of surgical life (and medicine more broadly) progressively deteriorate. Generally, the house of surgery has been unable or unwilling to push back against the rising tide of workplace nonsense and the subjugation of our colleagues to corporate and other special interests. Concern about the impact of this tedious and amoral performative environment, particularly on the well-being of our patients and young surgeons, has prevented me from disappearing entirely into the world of early bird dinners and bingo. I worry that our successors will think things were always this way and that this is the natural order of things.

It has been a custom of sorts to bemoan the perspectives, work habits and values of successive generations, especially in surgery. But my experience with the next generation of surgeons could not be more positive. I find young surgeons, residents and medical students to be extremely bright, deeply committed and altruistic. When I read the CV of applicants for surgery residency these days, I wonder if my achievements at a similar stage would be considered worth the price of a stamp on the application packet. I find their desire to have a work-life balance, treat all members of the healthcare team with respect and seek a diverse and inclusive environment to be refreshing.

If you are now rolling your eyes and expect me to continue on to the "politically correct," insincere delusional ramblings we are all so used to from leadership, don't worry. I will caution, however, that much of what is considered politically correct, I consider to be just plain correct. I believe what I said about these young surgeons. I hate what is happening to them and watching them be sold out, often without even knowing it. They deserve so much better.

Also, I must define a number of my baseline biases. Most contentious issues in this day and age seem to be addressed with mutually exclusive, competing narratives. But more than one thing can be true at the same time; truth is not a zero sum game. Having spent my entire career at two academic medical centers and having visited another 20-30 in a visiting professor capacity (yes, I am an old White guy with a picture), I do recognize the risks of overgeneralizing. It's true that if you know one place, you know one place.

But at every place that I have visited, there is a fundamental concern expressed about how the workplace is crushing the psyche of surgeons, especially early career surgeons. The utter ineptitude, ridiculousness and mind-numbing bureaucracy that continues to grow and flourish at "academic" medical centers and other healthcare delivery systems is bewildering and frustrating. The lack of a moral compass combined with the self-serving, performative behaviors so often in evidence in senior leadership, leave surgeons feeling devalued and lost. They work in a difficult environment without a sense of a shared mission.

In recent years, a few surgical leaders have attempted to move beyond the sterile euphemisms and timid, half-hearted efforts to confront tough issues such as burnout and the general failings of academic medical centers. These leaders deserve support and admiration; they have mine.

Speaking out (or failing to exhibit the expected degree of docile compliance) carries the risk of a surgeon not being considered a "team player" by their home institution. It is disappointing to see so many wink at leadership's counterfeit messaging and navigate around the basic values of the medical profession -- focusing instead on opportunities to game the system and exchange complicity for personal accolades and trophies.

I have thoroughly enjoyed my career and the years at the two academic medical centers where I worked. Although many things seemed wrongheaded and I have sometimes been passionate in calling them out, I am not an angry person and have no ax to grind. With maybe one or two exceptions, I have never worked with anyone I disliked personally. I am one of those people who really never personalizes anything. I cannot recall ever going home angry from work……not once.

I was extremely fortunate. I never felt "burned out" and always planned to step away in my mid-60s. I believe you sing your best song when you have the microphone and when it's time, step away on your own terms, graciously hand off the mic to the next person and leave the building. Don't linger around backstage. One of my senior colleagues once told me, "If you look in the mirror and see Dr. Hyman, don't retire. If you look in the mirror and see Neil, you will be fine." I am Neil.

I am a true believer in academic medicine. I just want us to do better and stop leading timidly from the rear. It is hurting our junior colleagues and the patients who rely on our integrity, fairness and respect for our social compact as professionals. As a profession, we are privileged with considerable autonomy in exchange for the expectation that we will place the needs of our patients and society first. I want us to be sure we earn and deserve that trust.

Further, I want to comment on style in the chapters ahead. Throughout my career, I tried to be sure all of my published work was faithfully referenced, precise and disciplined so as not to stray beyond the conclusions that could be fairly drawn from the data presented. As an editor, I have been a real pain in the ass about this expectation. Keep in mind that what follows are my reflections on a deteriorating healthcare environment and not a disciplined, evidence based manuscript.

I also do NOT want to call anyone out and intentionally will use blended or slightly amended emails and avoid using names/titles when I do have a criticism. I have no need to take any cheap shots at anyone as it is largely the system and culture that need to be fixed. I have no need or desire to demean anyone personally. So, if you feel in places that I am holding back, you are probably right.

Many of the e-mails included are the fifth, tenth or even twentieth in a series of communications aimed at solving a particular problem. As such, the tone is often strident or even sarcastic, reflecting my perceived need to shake things up, break through the lethargy and get someone's attention. This is not my preferred method of interaction and sincerely wish it was not so often necessary.

Lastly, I am, by nature, an informal person, which probably explains my career choice. Being a colorectal surgeon tends to protect against taking yourself too seriously. It is a wonderful specialty replete with outstanding people, broad-based commitment to the profession and the needs of patients and to each other as colleagues. I have worn a few different hats in academic medicine but never aspired to leadership per se. Over time, I accidentally learned that a little power can help you make good things happen for good people. It also gets you a seat at the few remaining tables where the perspective of the working clinician is included. My true loves were patient care, education, mentoring and research -- not administration. I never let that get out of balance.

I spent approximately 25 years on the faculty of the University of Vermont School of Medicine (UVM) and the last ~10 at the University of Chicago Pritzker School of Medicine (UChicago). They are both wonderful institutions in their own right with proud and rich traditions. I have many friends and colleagues at both places and have witnessed countless acts of generosity and kindness, as well as achievements that have advanced the field of surgery and medicine more generally. I have had the pleasure of working with many talented people of goodwill.

But truth be told, I cannot remember the last time I encountered a senior administrative leader driven by a commitment that is genuine, values-based and earnestly directed to societal needs. Virtually every administrative leadership meeting is all about maximizing revenue and issues are viewed primarily, if not entirely, through a financial prism. Healthcare has become strictly a business.

When I first started in surgery, I never would have believed that hospitals would advertise services and products like the manufacturers of skin moisturizers and that the primary goal would be to attract and preferentially provide care to those whose disease had the best reimbursement rate. Or that the needs of a community and "less desirable" sick people would be considered, at best, secondary and dismissed wherever performative messaging made it feasible.

I also do not want to take gratuitous cheap shots at leaders of modern healthcare institutions. My issues are not based on a Pollyanna view of the challenges. Indeed, if there is no money, there is no mission. Institutions must be run responsibly, capably and with fiscal discipline. My point is that the money really has become the mission. And the impact of the transition to healthcare as a business run by bureaucrats has been devastating for the well-being of surgeons and their patients.

We already have witnessed the impact of disenfranchising nurses with this approach, as they typically feel they have no leaders, no voice and are not being heard or valued. It feels like surgeons (and other physicians) are next. What does the future of healthcare look like if physicians and nurses feel entirely like "them" instead of "us" wherever they work?

Throughout my career and especially in recent years, I have met and worked with many surgeons. Their commitment, professionalism and dedication are truly outstanding -- everywhere I have been. Despite the ongoing decline in a sense of institutional mission, credible role models in leadership positions and the progressive invasion of suffocating bureaucracy, surgeons continue to do whatever is necessary to honor their professional commitment to their patients. How long can this last?

## THE BREAKING OF THE SURGEONS

Many surgeons have remarkable antipathy towards administrators. Despite the following criticisms, I generally do not. At both academic medical centers, I was a long-time division chief and co-led the Digestive Disease service line. Many administrators are also victimized by the system and perverse incentives that come down from the top. An inept, valueless and unproductive bureaucracy can rob anyone of meaning.

As a busy surgeon, I always knew that if I upset the wrong person in my modest administrative roles, I might have to go back to "just" being a doctor. That would have been perfectly fine. But the full-time administrator who doesn't play by the rules and "suck up" to the right people doesn't get promoted and may lose their job.

Quite often, administrators also want to have an impact and make things better for patients. But caution always is prudent, as taking initiative could be political suicide if it inadvertently undermined leadership and the self-serving rules of the C-suite. Protecting the status quo has made many senior leaders very, very rich.

# Chapter 1:
# The Way We Were

When I was a third-year medical student, a friend sent me *The Making of a Surgeon* by Dr. William Nolen. This book described Nolen's surgical residency at New York City's Bellevue Hospital in the 1960s and the excitement of surgical training. I was already considering a career in surgery; this book clinched the deal.

By the time I was a surgery resident in the mid-1980s at The Mount Sinai Medical Center in New York City, much had changed. Although we still had considerable autonomy, many of the "Wild West" aspects of the "see one, do one, teach one" approach had moderated to some extent in favor of more attending surgeon supervision and participation. The pyramid system had largely ended; this had been a competitive and potentially cutthroat system where a large group of residents would start together and each year some would be voted off the island until a select group remained to complete the program.

Although some rotations still were every other night on-call, most required "only" every third-night call. We were still working around 100-110 hours per week, the basic day being maybe 5:00 a.m. to 8:00 p.m. when not on call and then around 35-40 consecutive hours when you were. We almost always were exhausted and sleep-deprived. But we made enough money to pay rent and basic expenses. I remember my attendings claiming that they made $50 per month as a resident and had to wait tables the few nights they were not on call.

There was still pretty much no such thing as "abuse," as attending surgeons could largely say and do whatever they wanted to us. Profanity-laden criticisms, often quite personal and bellowed in public settings, were believed necessary to maintain discipline and ensure accountability. Physical abuse (e.g., forcefully whacking a resident's hands with heavy scissors during surgery) was still part of the "making of a surgeon."

Weekly morbidity conferences were showcases where residents expected to be belittled and shamed in front of their co-residents, medical students and the surgical staff. In fact, at many institutions, loosely affiliated or outside surgeons were invited to witness these spectacles and be impressed by how "tough" and "hard-nosed" the program and its leader really were. ANYTHING an attending surgeon told you to do was to be done faithfully; no questions asked.

One memorable example actually made its way into *The New York Times*. The Chair at one of the other major New York City teaching hospitals apparently had tried unsuccessfully for some time to get his residents to cut back on urinalyses, which overburdened the lab. He called a meeting. A warm substance resembling urine was poured into individual urine containers and placed in front of the senior residents. They were told to drink it. An excerpt from the article below details the incident.

### *THE DOCTOR'S WORLD; PRANK PUNISHES YOUNG SURGEONS (The New York Times,* September 4, 1984).

*One chief resident said he was not sure if there was urine in the containers when he put it to his lips. "We were unhappy about it and didn't feel we had much of a choice," said the resident, who asked that his name not be used. Another chief resident sipped from the container and then, realizing it was not the urine, chug-a-lugged the contents. The hazing ended the problem overnight. Word spread through the resident staff so quickly that not one urine sample was sent to the laboratory the next day.*

*The Department Chairman added, "People learn best by laughing or crying." He said the incident was part of the training of surgeons who must learn to do the routine almost as a drill so that they can act coolly in a medical crisis.*

*The laboratory director described the Chair as a "hero" for taking drastic action. He added, "Reductions in unnecessary testing do not come about unless there is continuous education…"*

This anecdote reflects the consensus thinking of the time and the training experience of surgeons in my generation. I doubt there are many who trained in the 1980s who would not be familiar with this mindset and approach to surgical training. It also helps, in retrospect, to illustrate how many things have changed for the better and not just for the worst, as many seem to contend. This type of "training" would almost be unimaginable now.

But I also view it as unfair when these stories are taken out of their time and context. Although sometimes misguided, I never had any doubt whatsoever during my training that the goal was to train me, build my character and prepare me for the rigors, accountability and professional obligations of a surgical career. The methods can and should be criticized; not necessarily the intent.

Further, not all of the surgeons were like this and, in fact, many were kind, showed that they cared about their trainees and took a clear interest in our futures. I had several wonderful role models and was exposed to a number of surgeons who took their responsibility for surgical education very seriously. To this day, like so many Mount Sinai residents who became colorectal surgeons, I considered Dr. Randy Steinhagen to be my primary role model when I was a surgery resident.

The Chairman of Mount Sinai's Department of Surgery was Dr. Arthur H. Aufses, Jr., a true gentleman with a leadership style that was quite atypical for that era. I first remember encountering Dr. Aufses at orientation for the surgery interns in 1984. Many of us relished our delusional identity as cool dudes and tended to wear our hair on the longer side. In the "boot camp" atmosphere era, where military discipline remained the order of the day in most surgical programs, we worried that he would make us all get military-style haircuts.

Although I had seen him before, my heart sank as he walked into the room with his ultrashort hair. About halfway through his rules of engagement speech, he said, "I choose to wear my hair like this. All I ask is that every day before you leave for work, you look in the mirror and imagine your grandmother is very sick and that someone who looks like you walks into the room to care for her. If you are satisfied, I will be satisfied." I never wanted to let him down -- my kind of leader.

As Dr. Nolen said, "The making of a surgeon is a tedious, painstaking, laborious and time-consuming process. The man who suffers through it will never forget it. I never have." Of course, that statement applies to women, too.

Indeed, passing on outrageous or heroic stories from one's training to the next generation, largely embellished and romanticized, continues to be a key component of the informal curriculum. I always have believed that I loved my years as a surgery resident. I really think I did, but it also seems possible that my memories are so distorted with the passing of time that they have become alternate reality memories… of great battles, heroic acts and the utter buffoonery of youth that have falsely become established as the official history and narrative. Who knows?

# THE BREAKING OF THE SURGEONS

We cherish these war stories and tend to share them anew at gatherings like combat veterans from the same platoon…over and over and over again…and more embellished each time. They preserve the bonds formed among those who trained together, cement the shared experience of those who have made it through surgical training and can have a welcoming or bonding effect with recent graduates or those who are in training. Shamefully, only in recent years have I wondered if everyone was really doing OK during training and what actually happened to the folks who started with us but did not finish.

It was also when I was a resident in New York that the Libby Zion fiasco occurred, planting the seeds for the development and implementation of resident work-hour restrictions. In brief, Libby Zion was a troubled young woman who was admitted to New York Hospital and died overnight, apparently from a drug interaction, now considered likely to have been serotonin syndrome. Her aggrieved father, who had been a prominent lawyer and written for several New York papers, including *The New York Times,* connected her death to an overworked intern and resident.

A civil trial and extensive media attention about the case lasted several years and Mr. Zion was even able to use his connections with the Manhattan District Attorney to convene a grand jury to assess if the house staff should be indicted for murder. One very clear and tangible result of all this attention was the creation of the Bell

Commission, which made assessments and recommendations about resident work-hour restrictions, which were implemented (or at least sort of implemented) in New York. Some have written that this event should be considered the "death" of American Medicine or "the end of the days of the giants."

Several spirited perspective pieces have been written about the Libby Zion incident. I have included a representative blog below by Dr Steven Knope (October 4, 1984, & Libby Zion: the day medicine changed forever) but I would urge you to read the many articles and perspectives that continue to appear to this day. Although I was training in New York as these events unfolded and experienced the early efforts to implement work-hour restrictions before they went national, I knew little of the case's many layers and nuances that existed behind the headlines. Given the number of hours we worked, pretty much anything (current and/or cultural events) that happened anywhere in the 1980s outside of Mount Sinai was a mystery to me.

*"Objectively, what caused the tragic death of Libby Zion was an arcane drug interaction between Nardil and Demerol. This drug interaction was virtually unknown by all doctors at the time, regardless of their level of training or experience....six medical department heads (Chiefs of Medicine at major hospitals) testified in the case. Several of these experts admitted under oath that they themselves had not heard of this drug interaction before the Zion*

*case. These men were among the most brilliant and esteemed physicians in the country.*

*Sidney Zion, the father of Libby Zion, was a wealthy and powerful attorney. He was also a former writer for the New York Times. He insisted that his daughter had died due to overwork and a lack of supervision of these young doctors. Sidney Zion went public and began to refer to his daughter's death in The New York Times as a 'murder.' The untenable argument made by Mr. Zion was that if only an attending physician had been in the hospital, if only these young doctors had been better supervised or more rested, his daughter would still be alive.*

*The effect this case had on the training of doctors cannot be overemphasized. Doctors today see less disease during a critical point in their training than they used to. They lose continuity of care by having to leave sick patients during critical points in their illnesses. This has also changed young doctors' attitudes about their professional identity. They no longer expect to take complete ownership of the care of their patients. They see themselves as part of a team, as opposed to the professional who is primarily responsible for human life."*

Although many of our internal medicine colleagues were in favor of work-hour restrictions, every single one of the surgery residents I knew was adamantly against them. Many resented the irrational and seemingly unwarranted intrusion of the government and political hacks into our training. Some were deeply offended that this well-connected trial lawyer could make use of his political friends and connections to unjustly and cruelly bully the besieged medical residents who had cared for his daughter; and even continue to publicly label his daughter's tragic death as "murder" and the intern and resident as "murderers."

But above all, we just did not want to be forced to walk away and leave our patients, especially the sickest ones, who we felt needed us. If ANYTHING was repugnant and repulsive to our professional identity, it was that. Of no surprise to most of us, work-hour restrictions have not made care safer and it is hard to argue that there were any direct or even indirect benefits to patient safety.

Nonetheless, I was an early advocate of the *concept* of work restrictions and think it was and is the right thing to do. It was really the implementation of the restrictions and the program leadership's frequent inability to think outside the box that was often the problem. The approach was to try and load all of the cargo from the old school bus into the new minivan. Eighty hours a week for five years is a lot of time. Back then, I believed and still believe that if we cannot train the very best and brightest of their generation to do what we do in that time span, the fault really should be with us/our educational system and not the time constraints.

Way too much time is wasted and we routinely fail to make education a priority, throwing trainees under the bus with a continuous stream of work with little or no educational value, succumbing to administrators' voracious appetite for forms and bureaucracy. Residents are easily accessed and burdened with "scut" work by almost anyone in the system, as they have little voice and are only "passing through" the institution.

No one pulled my sons out of social studies class in high school because the janitor did not show up and someone needed to take out the garbage from the cafeteria. But iterative work rains down on our residents in training from many directions and their educational needs are not adequately valued and protected. Education has turned out to be the poor stepchild just about everywhere in academic medicine and remains an ongoing failure of surgical leadership.

## Chapter 2:
## The Fantasy Football League

I love sports. I grew up in New York as a die-hard Giants, Yankees, Knicks and initially Rangers then Islanders fan. Unqualified devotion to these teams (well, at least the Giants, Yankees and Islanders) probably was the only mandatory condition for our two sons to live in our house.

As a kid, I loved collecting baseball and football cards. I would sit on the floor of the room I shared with my brother and build teams with the cards. OK, I just got a Dave Robinson card and I can put him as an outside linebacker next to Dick Butkus in the middle. I would construct my team and think about my next pack of cards. What if I got a Bobby Bell? Who would start on my team: Robinson or Bell? Would I keep Robinson in on running plays and then bring Bell in on third and long? How did my team compare to the teams my buddies on the block had? I could occupy my mind for hours reconfiguring my team and actually felt some satisfaction with my shrewd moves in this imaginary world.

My grown sons and their friends do the same sort of thing with their fantasy football leagues. They create lineups by selecting players in a draft from any team in the NFL and accumulate points to defeat their rival's imaginary team. When they win games in this alternative reality world, they congratulate themselves on their football knowledge and insights. They make weekly decisions of who to "play" based on the projected number of points for the players on their make-believe roster. Mainstream sports entertainment shows actually provide expert advice and opinion each week on these fantasy leagues.

But everyone understands that the fantasy football league is not reality. Real games are played on the field with real points, touchdowns, field goals, fumbles and interceptions. There are remarkable individual feats of athleticism and character, strategies based on careful preparation and success based on committed teamwork. There is no escape from the final score and personal accountability. The real players go home with injuries, pain and mud on their uniforms.

There is no recognized distinction between the fantasy football league and reality in the C-suites of many healthcare organizations. Healthcare leaders and administrators have so profoundly insulated themselves from the nuances and challenges of patient care and may have so little familiarity with the clinical enterprise, that they have created a fantasy football league equivalent that they manage as if it were reality -- all while sequestered in the luxury boxes high above and removed from the playing field (the hospital, clinics and operating rooms), where the real game is played. In this healthcare fantasy football league, virtual or imaginary problems are defined, processes and solutions crafted based on magical data. There are ever fewer folks among the increasingly crowded cliques in the luxury boxes who have any idea what is actually going on. And somehow, this is not considered a problem.

This trend really crossed another threshold during the COVID-19 pandemic when administrators and leadership largely worked remotely. It used to be that bonafide physician leaders were viewed as indispensable to understanding the problems and challenges that patients and care providers experience. Now, there's often no one to call out the oblivious chatter in the C-suite and distinguish it from the lived reality on the playing field. The make-believe data and reports shared in this fantasy football league have become the *de facto* operational reality.

Healthcare organizations have devolved into two parallel universes of people: one group sits in the luxury boxes and the other works on the field. With the exponential growth of people crowding into the box, it becomes harder to see the field (and some in the box are heavily invested in blocking the view and making sure the blinds are down). It is the virtual reality of the fantasy football league where leadership accumulates points, transactional relationships are built, promotions are decided and mega dollar, baseball-type contracts are increasingly awarded.

Healthcare workers tend to think that folks in the C-suite, by virtue of their specialized language and business training, can solve operational problems. In most organizations, they cannot; they don't understand them. Physicians look up into the boxes and assume that the leaders are seeing the game on the field and are aware of the fundamental nature of the challenges they experience. Often, this could not be further from the truth.

Since those in the boxes typically do not deliver care to patients and many never have, they are unable to understand the substance or context of the data provided to them. As such, typically, they are unable to make thoughtful decisions that impact patient care unless they have earnest, energized and respectful partnerships with legitimate physician leaders. Otherwise, the luxury box attendees remain unaware that they are leading a fantasy football team rather than the real thing.

Senior leaders are commonly unable to recognize when data is faulty (or even made up) and they are led astray easily. It is for this reason that physician-administrator partnerships are so important in getting it right. These teams have largely disappeared in many organizations, as the physician at the table is now increasingly what I call a PINO (Physician In Name Only). Somehow, it is assumed that a physician is knowledgeable, insightful and experienced in the patient care challenges of that particular institution based on an M.D. degree, even if they have never provided patient care at that institution or anywhere else for that matter. It is concluded that an MBA, rather than actual experience practicing medicine, best meets the leadership needs of the organization.

In fairness, there are a handful of major healthcare organizations led quite successfully by experienced, insightful and highly competent surgeons/physicians. These organizations are typically the ones that are successful and high-functioning. Again, if you know one place, you know one place.

However, faulty context-free analyses provided to the unaware have major impacts on organizational effectiveness. For the working surgeon, the cumulative impact of uninformed leadership can feel more like death by a thousand cuts. Will these leaders ever do anything meaningful that makes sense? For example, I was called into a luxury box when I was Chief of General Surgery at UVM and walked into a room filled with grim faces. It was explained to me that a committee had been formed under the auspices of a PINO to assess surgical complications, as there was an awareness from one of the healthcare management journals that complications were costly.

At UVM, under Dr. Steve Shackford's leadership, we had a VERY robust and accountable quality system and culture and I found it very unlikely that the group in the luxury box would bring up something substantive. I was told that a group (no surgeon included) had been meeting weekly for a year and had discovered that there was a "surgeon" on staff who had a 100% anastomotic leak rate (a leak which can occur when two pieces of intestine are joined together). Obviously, this was ludicrous and I couldn't wait to find out how this "revelation" had been uncovered. Our Department internally tracked the leak rate of all surgeons in real-time and I could usually quote the data from memory.

As a born and bred curmudgeon with poor tolerance for the PowerPoint excesses of the luxury boxes, for once I managed to sit quietly through the parade of meaningless "filler" slides, hoping that the next one would finally be the one with actual content. At the meeting, everyone involved was introduced, their background reviewed, they were all congratulated, and the word "transparent" was used on just about every slide. As the PowerPoint meandered along, finally, on slide 51, the name of the "surgeon" in question was revealed. It was a pulmonologist from the Medical Intensive Care Unit, who, of course, is not a surgeon and does not do intestinal surgery, let alone perform anastomoses.

I was amazed that a project like this could go on for a year and no one seemed to think that legitimate expertise would help. I smugly asked how many anastomoses this physician had performed. No one in the room knew the answer or the physician's specialty. It turns out that there had been two patients transferred to UVM for critical care after a leak from surgery at another hospital and the physician of record was the admitting intensivist. No surgery had been performed at UVM. Yet again, the clueless playing make-believe and performing in a vacuum.

The physician-administrator partnership has become way out of balance. Physician "leaders" are often just middle managers. They commonly agree to do the bidding/messaging of the administrative leaders so they can enjoy the prestige and benefits of their position. This diminished role is particularly acute in many academic medical centers, where the healthcare system or hospital is often academic in name only. Titles are showered on surgeons who may have almost no power just so the basic facade of an academic structure can be simulated.

It was not always this way. When I started at UVM, the hospital president would eat lunch with staff almost every day in the cafeteria. He used to join us at our table and ask how things were going and what we needed. There were very few administrators back then (a tiny fraction of what we have now -- much more about that later) and most key decisions were made in partnership with department chairs. We were all on the same team; we were "us." Highly respected and accomplished physicians led the organization and the Chiefs of Medicine and Surgery were the most powerful positions in the hospital.

By training and professional norms, physicians and nurses have somewhat different values than administrators. But I do not think it is fair to claim that administrators are by nature the heartless and soulless boogeymen/women that physicians like to talk about in the doctor's lounge. By the nature of our respective jobs, patients appear to administrative leaders as data files in aggregate -- yet to a physician or nurse, they are our individual patients. We know them personally and often intimately and share their successes and/or pain firsthand. Adverse decisions cause harm to someone we care about, not to a spreadsheet.

This is why the formal communication that comes down from the luxury boxes usually appears tone-deaf. Leaders who seem to know absolutely nothing about what is really going on rely on a communications expert to message the care providers, who live the actual reality every day. The mass-produced email is typically a generic/empty boilerplate, performative expression of appreciation that screams insincerity and has no basis in reality (e.g., everything here is perfect, only getting better and we have everything under control). Most physicians and nurses want to feel like part of the team and not be relentlessly patronized. We want honest and meaningful communication rather than insincere platitudes produced by a communications team under the signature of a leader. That approach would seem appropriate when one wants to treat folks as "them" and not "us."

Just the language of the luxury box is a real morale killer. Although I always spent the great majority of time throughout my career as a working physician, I most often had leadership positions that would necessitate visits to the luxury boxes. A visit to the box had its benefits: always plenty of food and refreshments, never any problem securing the nicest meeting room and no need to be available any time of day or night for the meeting (unlike surgeons waiting for operating room availability).

I am not claiming that healthcare leaders are stupid or incompetent. I do not believe them to be fundamentally evil or uncaring. They just don't know what they don't know and, at this point, have no reason to view that as a problem. They have systematically indoctrinated the healthcare team with a language full of empty and insincere euphemisms.

The separation of administration from those who deliver care takes many forms: physical, values-based, communication, language and even financial. All of these merit comments. First, the C-suite is usually well separated geographically from the care areas; leaders do not see the day-to-day bustle and problems encountered where the nurses, physicians and other healthcare providers struggle to provide optimal patient care. I remember the CEO at UVM walking to the C-suite every day through the underground tunnels, presumably to avoid the risk of running into the medical staff. Further, there are now so many tiers of management (especially in nursing) that one has to go down many, many layers of the organizational chart before encountering someone who touches a patient. As a result, decisions often have no basis in reality, as no one at the table knows what the reality is. And in the healthcare version of the fantasy football league, there is no source of truth to contend with.

## THE BREAKING OF THE SURGEONS

There was a monumental shift in UVM's Department of Surgery when our Chair Steve Shackford left. Highly principled, "Shack" held us strictly accountable to the key tenets of professionalism and our social compact: we put our patients first and worked as a team. We always knew what our values were and had a shared sense of mission. If you believed academic medicine was only about you, you could leave. It was fun going to work. Morale was high, we had each other's back and there was a very real personal and professional camaraderie.

But then came the underground CEO, who clearly did not see us as partners or teammates and viewed our cohesiveness as a threat to the docile conformity expected from "the help." Without Shack, we lost our leader, our voice and our sense of belonging. Other key leaders in the department soon headed for the door as it became increasingly clear that the traditional values of academic medicine and professionalism were considered outdated relics of an earlier time. The PINO (Physician In Name Only) approach was to be the coin of the realm. Lip service to the academic mission was the Dean's job. Physicians would focus strictly on coding, billing and the bottom line…and staying quiet. No need to be bothered with the pesky issues of high-quality, responsive patient care; creating appearances for the Board of Trustees and regulators would be more than sufficient.

## THE BREAKING OF THE SURGEONS

One nice illustration of the changes in the environment in the "post Shackford" era was the vacation policy conflict. When Shack became Chair in 1989, he moved the Department more towards a specialized surgical practice model rather than a generalist "everyone does everything" approach. One challenge in a relatively small department in a rural state like Vermont was making sure there was adequate coverage for subspecialties that might have had only one surgeon.

When I came to UVM in 1990, I was the first and only fellowship-trained colon and rectal surgeon in either Vermont or New Hampshire. Of course, there had been highly skilled surgeons doing colon and rectal cases for many years. But prior to my arrival, the most complicated IBD (inflammatory bowel disease) cases and rectal reconstructions typically were sent to the Lahey clinic outside of Boston. I was trained to do those cases and appreciated the opportunity and privilege to care for these patients.

When I was away at a conference or on vacation, Vermonters might have to make the trip down to Boston. Shack did not prevent me from taking a vacation or going to meetings, but he asked that I try to be available to referring GI docs by phone when away (e.g., for patients with severe, medically refractory colitis), to help get patients transferred in and to limit my vacation time for the first few years until the specialized surgical practice program was established.

## THE BREAKING OF THE SURGEONS

These unused vacation days would be banked and either used later or "cashed out" at retirement, a notoriously unproductive time for surgeons. Surgeons do not consider it prudent to take on new patients and major cases just before retiring and/or leaving the institution. This was a real win for UVM. The idea was that once the program was successful and the numbers justified it, the department would hire another colon and rectal surgeon. Indeed, several years later, we did just that; there were four fellowship-trained colon and rectal surgeons at UVM by the time I left in 2014.

Like a number of the handful of specialty surgeons who had banked vacation days, I had donated most of them to the UVM medical center in support of a capital campaign (the Renaissance Project), leaving me with a modest number of days in the bank. Years later, when another Shackford era surgeon was planning to leave, we discussed donating our remaining days to the institution in support of residency training. Dr. Dennis Vane had been the Vice Chair in the Department for Clinical Affairs and, for many years, had been the only pediatric surgeon in Vermont, taking all of the night and weekend calls for years.

Out of the blue, we were notified that the vacation day balances would not be honored. For me, it was not really a major financial issue as I had donated many of the days. I was one of the last holdovers from the Shackford era and suspected we were just being targeted to kick sand in our face, as a demonstration of power and message to the other surgeons. I could not imagine any moral or rational justification for such a sleazy move.

I brought this concern to Shack's replacement and he would just say that he had been instructed not to honor the commitment. I asked him and a number of other senior leaders, including the hospital attorney, simply to provide some sort of justification or explanation. They would not or could not. Ultimately, Dennis and I agreed to arbitration to settle the issue. To this day, I don't have any idea what really happened behind the scenes in the luxury boxes. Truth can be virtually impossible to get from senior administrative leadership. It is perceived as having little or no value and even dangerous. Instead, "messaging" is always the coin of the realm.

In retrospect, these events ushered in the fantasy football league era at UVM. There would not be the same partnership with physicians; healthcare was a business to be run by "professionals" and surgeons would need to keep their advocacy of the values of their profession and the academic medical center to themselves. Professional values and the tripartite missions of education, research and clinical innovation largely would instead be simulated by those on the medical school side, where they developed another set of compensatory magical thinking. The Dean and academic leaders could feel free to make all the speeches they wanted at an endless array of ceremonies. But that activity was for show; the CEO controlled the finances and the goal was to make the surgeons run on the treadmill as fast as they could to make money for the luxury box inhabitants.

Shortly before I left UVM and moved to the University of Chicago, a highly respected surgeon was brought in to lead the practice group and replace the previous leader, who also was a surgeon by training. His predecessor had been a PINO who we barely knew as he chose not to interact much with the "regular" surgeons engaged in clinical medicine. The new faculty practice leader clearly seemed to be a good man and had been well-liked by surgeons I knew and trusted. Dr. Marion Couch had become Interim Chair and had done well in that role: restoring a sense of basic dignity and kinship in the Department. I liked and respected Marion very much. After an unsuccessful search for a permanent Chair (which, amazingly, the Dean explicitly characterized as "successful" -- no candidate offered the job accepted it, so no one "bad" was chosen), Dr. Mitch Norotsky was selected Interim Chair and subsequently named permanent Chair.

Mitch was a junior resident when I arrived at UVM and I am very fond of him. I only provide this information as background to the letter written below to the new leader of the faculty practice. There were looming financial issues and we had recently received horrid results from a physician satisfaction survey that was being suppressed by leadership. I had gone before the Board of Trustees earlier when Shack's successor was Chair and things were really bottoming out. I felt I owed this to my junior colleagues as one of the last ones standing from the Shackford era. At that time, the University of Vermont Medical Center was known as Fletcher Allen Healthcare (FAHC). Believe it or not, they had paid a consulting firm big bucks for that name. And ironically, the new slogan was "Becoming One," as if a slogan alone would engage physicians.

*Dear Dr. X,*

*I just thought I would send this to you on background: 3 years ago (2011), after many, many unsuccessful efforts to get an "audience" with senior leadership and as more and more of our high-performing and talented department leaders left (and fear/anxiety levels grew to an astounding level among our younger guys), I could no longer sit idly by. I went before the Board of Trustees and read the statement below. As expected, this is when I went from a "golden boy" in the department to a "bad apple" in the eyes of senior leadership.*

*Obviously, with the steady hand and unshakable integrity of Marion's leadership, much has improved. As you know from our discussion, I strongly support Mitch as well and believe he was absolutely the right choice to carry the ball at this point. But I would focus you on the last paragraph of the statement where I point out the inevitable effect on surgical productivity and revenue-I know this can sometimes be the only way to get senior leadership's attention.*

## THE BREAKING OF THE SURGEONS

*When one considers that almost all of our leaders have left or been disenfranchised and that we have developed no one to take their place (this cannot happen in an environment where communication is unidirectional and there are limited or no opportunities for surgeons to control their work environment), progressive inefficiency and malaise are inevitable. If one then adds the ineffectiveness and inefficiency of the OR, we have a perfect storm. At one point, I think we had 6 nurse leaders in 7 years, and the position has been vacant at times as well -- most recently for almost a year.*

*In short, I really do not believe we will be able to turn the volume issue around unless we deal with the work environment, build a team approach based on mutual respect, and create a collaborative spirit where surgeons believe their personal and professional fate is linked to that of the institution. I feel confident that surgeons who believe they are valued and respected will be more productive. See below from 2011.*

*Many thanks*

*Neil*

Members of the Board of Trustees,

I would like to express my gratitude to the Board for this opportunity. My name is Neil Hyman, and I've been a surgeon here for 21 years. I have come to address the progressive deterioration in *physician morale that has resulted in a seriously dissatisfied, disenfranchised, and ominously disengaged medical staff. I'm sure you understand the consequences this has for the overall work climate, physician retention, recruitment, and, ultimately the quality of care we deliver to our patients. The issues of morale and dissatisfaction, at least in Surgery, are now known throughout the country; we have quickly gone from a desirable medical community to a "red-flagged" hotbed of discontent and adversarial relationships. Our problems have become a subject of local and national attention.*

*I am uncertain if the administration is out of touch and they don't know what's behind the dissatisfaction or if they simply hope to ignore it. Administrative efforts to "perfume the pig" with slogans and cosmetic initiatives are perceived as insulting or frankly degrading by many. Physicians may be averse to conflict, but we are intelligent human beings. Almost any physician here can tell you what the fundamental problems are. They are not complex, and the perceptions and causes of discontent are broadly shared and very well known. But we all have families to support and careers to build. If you walk the halls, you will often see physicians whispering in the shadows, looking around the corner for who is watching and being careful who they are seen talking to.*

*I was originally on the physician satisfaction committee that administrated the survey; a major problem we had was convincing physicians that the survey really was anonymous and untraceable. We were told by a number of physicians that they were afraid to fill out the form because they "had heard" that FAHC could track the responses.*

*The management strategy is perceived as containment: marginalize, threaten, and punish those who speak up. For this reason, I sheepishly mention that I have been Teacher of the Year in the College of Medicine three times, served for many years on the medical staff executive committee, and was recently named Physician of the Year by the Vermont State Medical Society. I am no outlier. I have never sought a leadership position at FAHC and cherish my relationship with my coworkers; I have dedicated my career to this place. Among the most difficult aspects is the alienation of our support staff. Many of them have lived in Vermont their whole lives and have worked only for FAHC. Their connection and loyalty to FAHC is a critical part of their identity. The dissatisfaction is hardly a medical staff issue alone. At the end of the day, our academic medical center does not belong to me, the physicians or the administrative inner circle; it belongs to the people of Vermont who rely on us to do right by them.*

*In the 2009 survey, the national norm for overall satisfaction was 36% "highly satisfied" for surgeons in academic medical centers; at FAHC, this number was 0%. Conversely, 9% of surgeons elsewhere described themselves as somewhat or very dissatisfied; at*

*FAHC, this number was 47%. There was no action taken, no discussion, and no sign of interest from senior leadership. In the 2010 survey, 84% of FAHC surgeons were dissatisfied with the communication from leadership, 89% were dissatisfied with institutional morale, and 80% felt they did not have input into the practice group policies. This was the 0th percentile nationally and probably the very worst results of any institution in the United States. You can't successfully intimidate and marginalize 89% of the physicians. So what is going on?*

*First, senior leadership does not appear interested in gaining our confidence or trust. We do not really know any of these people except by distorted caricature; they seem oddly disconnected from our core business-patient care. I can recall Dr. Y coming to our Department meetings twice over the last few years. In a Dept. with over 90 members at last count, there were less than ten people who thought it worthwhile to hear the CEO.*

*Let me address one specific issue in my limited time -- the lingering vacation policy conflict, that was addressed with the Board two years ago by several of my colleagues.*

*When I came here in 1990, I was the first and only colorectal surgeon. Dr. Shackford asked that I limit my vacation days as he did for others with a unique skill set since reliable access is a critical ingredient in building a new clinical program. As compensation, he would allow us to bank these days and use them when we left FAHC;*

*for surgeons, this wind-down time is notoriously unproductive. Many of the procedures I had been trained to do were only available in Boston. For my first ten years here, I almost invariably made rounds seven days a week and was accessible at virtually all times, often even while on vacation. We now have three busy colorectal surgeons, and a business plan is being developed for a fourth. In 2001, I donated a large number of my days to FAHC in support of the Renaissance Project, leaving me with a rather modest balance.*

*In February of 2008, a rumor started circulating that our vacation balances would not be respected. Most of us understood that the new Chair could have any policy he wanted going forward but did not consider that the previously tracked, reported, and audited days would be invalidated unilaterally. As such, we were very surprised later in the month when we received an opinion letter from Mr. Z indicating that he did not believe FAHC had a legal obligation to honor the promise.*

*I met with Dr. X and explained that I never had the intention of asking to be paid for the days, even though I believed it was my right. However, I did not understand how FAHC could simply refuse to honor a Chair's openly disclosed policy that they knew about for many years, which was described in a 2001 Price Waterhouse Coopers audit, an internal FAHC audit, and numerous internal documents over the years. It was common knowledge among senior leadership. He told us repeatedly that Dr Y and Mr Z had "tied his hands" or "instructed that I can neither pay nor budget the liability" or "had prohibited him" from honoring the promise which Dr Shackford explained had been made in good faith, benefitted FAHC and which we relied on; the fundamental trust that is required in the workplace was profoundly undermined.*

*Two of us filed for arbitration to defend against what we perceived to be pure bullying.*

*The arbitrator ruled that we were entitled to half of the cash value of our excess vacation days; this about paid for my legal expenses. FAHC's counsel sent a letter to the other 26 surgeons with balances expressing great satisfaction with the outcome, yet quietly submitted a motion to modify the findings. At the end of the day, they preferred to spend hundreds of thousands of FAHC dollars in legal fees rather than talk to me. The Vermont Superior Court upheld the arbitrators award without modification.*

*How does the CEO and hospital attorney prohibiting our Chairman from honoring an acknowledged promise or instructing him not to do so facilitate "Becoming One?" Even if FAHC somehow believed their actions were morally justifiable, why wouldn't you at least be willing to have a dialogue with the other members of the Department who this affects once the arbitrator ruled and the motion to modify was rejected? How is this "becoming one?" Why is this allowed to fester like an open wound?*

## THE BREAKING OF THE SURGEONS

*Physicians have a professional obligation and oath to advocate for our patients. As our senior people continue to leave, we will have a harder and harder time recruiting talented physicians to our ranks, and eventually we will become a second rate institution. You may have observed that our surgical volumes have already started to decline. I expect the healthcare environment to grow more challenging in the years ahead, and we need to all be on the same page; led with integrity and a unified sense of mission. We need to be inspired or at least respected rather than dismissed. We need to feel that we work for an institution that has a moral compass, shared values and respects the fundamental rights and dignity of its employees. An academic medical center works best as a democratic institution where the tension between the interests of the various constituencies and the competing missions drives dialogue based on mutual respect. The satisfaction issue is all of our problem and responsibility to work on together.*

# Chapter 3:
# On Activity, Achievement and the Clipboard Nurses

This seems like a good time to reiterate the aim of this book. Except perhaps for a very short period of time described in the last chapter, I appreciated my time at UVM. There were so many good people there. I worked with excellent surgeons, the nurses were wonderful and the residents/medical students were just terrific. I always felt that I had just about the best job in the world and had never considered leaving.

In my almost 25 years at UVM, I had never gone on another job interview or even taken a phone call to discuss a new opportunity. But as a surgeon with a longstanding interest in inflammatory bowel disease, when UChicago came calling, I felt ready to consider a move. I always have been extraordinarily fortunate throughout my career to be happy and appreciate my circumstances. Despite being a pain in the ass who will speak out when I think things are unfair and unjust, I cannot remember once going home angry or with a perceived need for retribution or a sense of grievance. How lucky is that….

Rather, I intend to illustrate how the fantasy football league and bunker mentality of senior leadership have made the lives of surgeons (and physicians and nurses more broadly) much less satisfying, more difficult and have undermined the sense of teamwork and belonging that is so crucial to a successful healthcare organization. Although my focus is on surgeons, as that's what I know best, the same or similar things could be said about any other category of healthcare provider. The natural history of fantasy football league/alternative reality management on patient safety, quality outcomes and staff retention is obvious and it is only getting worse.

Different perceptions of reality can create division and mutual antipathy between those sitting in the luxury boxes and those working on the playing field. But one should never attribute to malice that which is attributable to ignorance. I believe this is derived from Hanlon's razor, which states, "never attribute to malice that which is adequately explained by stupidity." Although more cumbersome, Douglas W. Hubbard in his 2020 book, *The Failure of Risk Management: Why it's broken and how to fix it*, rephrased Hanlon's razor as "never attribute to malice or stupidity that which can be explained by moderately rational individuals following incentives in a complex system."

Examining what has happened over the past 30 years in nursing is particularly instructive. I respect nurses and like most surgeons (or at least those with any sense), appreciate that they are the backbone of patient care. When I started practice, the basic care model was bedside nurses led by a respected, experienced and knowledgeable nurse manager who had an office on the floor. Nurse managers were invaluable resources to patients and surgical trainees, and as problem-solvers and mentors to other nurses. If one of the surgery residents acted disrespectfully to one of the nurses, I would hear about it from the nurse manager (and make sure the offender made the obligatory trip to the woodshed). Healthcare is a team sport and this type of behavior cannot be tolerated. If there were issues impacting patient care, the head nurse would catch me on rounds and tell me. In those days, a surgeon usually could just fix the problems; there used to be MUCH more camaraderie and teamwork between physicians and nurses.

Then came the proliferation of what we came to call the "clipboard nurses." Nurses with advanced degrees (sometimes with very limited clinical experience and little or no familiarity with the institutional culture and practice) would direct nursing from a remote site. Periodically, a group of five or six would appear, clipboard in hand, in a patient care area. They would write a few things on a clipboard and stare at one of the floor nurses taking care of a patient. The clipboard nurse often would try to figure out what the nurse was doing (and once in a while even put the clipboard down and awkwardly try to help without appearing foolish).

Soon, the clipboard nurses would generate a new set of forms and add them to the ever-expanding documentation burden the floor nurses needed to complete for every patient every day. Quite often, the same repetitive information already was being captured on other forms (because communication between the clipboard pods was so poor) and no one really could say how the data would be used. With the EMR (electronic medical record), this typically amounts to nurses copying and pasting the same partially completed form on the patient every day. Lather, rinse, repeat, over and over again for many years and you have a system where nurses spend the bulk of their day completing mindless paperwork at a bank of computers at the nursing station or outside a patient's room. And then they are unable to do what they love: caring for patients.

The phenomenon of nurse leaders separating and sequestering themselves from the bedside nurses became endemic before this separation trended on the physician side. Today it's even worse as the "clipboard" is electronic and there is little or no perceived reason for the clipboard nurses actually to visit the patient care areas. They don't see what is happening or talk with the bedside nurses. Communication is almost exclusively through shallow and impersonal emails.

When I made rounds years back, the head nurse and/or the nurse caring for a patient would join me if they were free to make sure we were all on the same page and that all of the patient's needs and concerns were addressed (e.g., "Remember Ms. Smith, you wanted to ask Dr. Hyman if you would be able to make that trip to visit your children in Ohio next month"). Now, if I ask a nurse, "How is Ms.

Smith doing today?" they usually look at me blankly. I have learned I need to ask, "How is bed 65-2 doing today?" Owing to documentation requirements and "top-down," remote leadership, nurses may spend almost their entire shift on the computer, completing documentation requirements with limited direct patient contact. This is not their fault, nor does it reflect their compassion or professionalism. In fact, nurses hate it and complain about it all the time. They are as wonderful and committed as ever.

Similarly, in the OR, I always had enjoyed the partnership with nursing and/or the scrub tech; so many times their useful suggestions, observations and attention saved the patient and me from a potential adverse event. Now, the circulating nurse and even the scrub tech may not look at the operative field once during an entire case. Instead, they spend their time charting mountains of irrelevant minutia and signing out to a relief nurse who seems to appear every 20-30 minutes. The staff seldom asks about the patient, the goals of the operation, the next steps, etc. At the end of the operation, they often do not know what operation we performed or what we removed and why. Contributing to the safety and well-being of the patient takes a back seat to documentation and participation in the team is often limited to completing forms. This is not professionally fulfilling and it makes nurses leave the institution for the highest bidder or nursing altogether.

## THE BREAKING OF THE SURGEONS

It just does not suffice for the Chief Nursing Officer to make an annual appearance on the wards the day before Thanksgiving to deliver a turkey. In this now familiar scenario, a team of escorts arrives with a photographer in tow so the blessed event can be captured for the newsletter. Very few of the nurses ever met the CNO and most have never seen her/him in the hospital. To believe this annual showcase will convince rank-and-file nurses that the CNO understands them, the challenges they experience or has their back is ludicrous. But this performance works just fine in the fantasy football league.

Nurses are every bit as dedicated as they were 30 years ago. They are thoughtful, caring, skilled and work very hard. However, the expectation of meaningful participation is undermined by the clipboard nurse and nursing leadership culture, who are focused from afar exclusively on something else (budgets, staffing). The pervasive infestation of paperwork, forms and charting that characterizes modern nursing deprives these wonderful and committed professionals of the personal joy and meaning that is so important to their well-being, team performance, and most importantly, patient care. As we have seen in recent years, this paperwork frenzy has been a disaster for nursing retention and burnout. This should serve as a cautionary tale for healthcare leaders regarding what's coming with their surgeons and medical staff.

## THE BREAKING OF THE SURGEONS

When I arrived at UChicago, many things were fundamentally different from UVM, again highlighting that if you know one place, you know one place. This is why I acknowledge that one must be cautious about broad generalizations. I have no doubt that many of my comments and illustrations provided do not reflect the successes that many healthcare organizations achieve. But I do think it is very clear that progressive marginalization and loss of empowerment among surgeons is ubiquitous and threatens the future of healthcare delivery. Generally, the examples I provide are site-specific but do represent an overarching trend with ominous implications.

When I was recruited to UChicago, there was a clear and universal appreciation expressed for the pervasive operational deficits and challenges. There were world-class researchers and clinicians; there still are. But things like answering phones, arranging appointments, facilitating patient access and care integration were woefully deficient. This was readily acknowledged by just about everyone in leadership. I was being brought in, along with others, to help change this deeply entrenched culture of malaise and disabling ineffectiveness.

As opposed to an ever-increasing number of "academic medical centers" where the CEO/hospital president has all the money and the dean of the medical school walks around with tin cup in hand, the Dean at UChicago was the boss. And as a true believer in the mission and traditional values of the academic medical center, I really liked this arrangement. But I also believe that medical professionals need to put patient and community needs front and center. Excelling in research does not have to be a choice that precludes responsiveness to patient needs. Providing high-quality, compassionate care does not make a research portfolio less impressive.

I also do not respect arrogance and those who use their leadership position primarily for personal gain. Especially at an academic medical center, the fundamental goals and mission of faculty must include serving as role models and mentors for medical students/trainees and fostering the future success of our junior colleagues. It's unsettling how many academic physicians take a position of leadership primarily to arrange to win trophies and see their portrait on a wall someday.

Physicians were welcomed in the room where it happens or at least faithfully included in key committees and initiatives. Probably because the Dean ran the organization (as opposed to an administrator or PINO), there were physician leaders in leadership. The problem was that many of these physicians insulated themselves from the rank and file, zealously protected their positions, controlled information and generally maintained the status quo at all costs.

Physician leadership positions at UChicago are justifiably prestigious. There are considerations of legacy, opportunities for national and international leadership, recognition and acclaim. Folks do not tend to give up these privileges easily. It is perhaps predictable that dealing with the more mundane and grinding issues of operational effectiveness, efficiency and patient care are considered beneath them. The primary focus for too many is on personal advancement and one quickly learns that many will preferentially bullshit their way through situations and strive to wallpaper over operational problems to avoid being exposed.

But it is difficult for a healthcare system seeking to compete and succeed if it openly ignores service and responsive patient care. This is EXACTLY why the alternative reality of fantasy football became so attractive for many in leadership. The nuances, inconvenient truths and constant attention to detail required for excellence in actual care settings can be substituted with smoke and mirror reports, perfunctory data files and the empty language of the administrative world. The constant hum of this activity and counterfeit work provides a sense that the institution is professionally managed. The status quo is preserved, no one loses their position and no one is forced to "waste time" on the arcane and work-intensive challenges patient care demands.

Iconic UCLA basketball coach John Wooden is often quoted as having said, "Never mistake activity for achievement." In my wildest dreams, I had never imagined an organization where the ratio of activity to achievement was so high. The same operational issues would be addressed over and over again. After a couple of years, I knew the routine quite well. A committee would be formed in the name of "inclusion" that was way too large to get anything done. There could be easily 50-100 people involved. The committee almost never had a clear charge and there never seemed to be any specific deliverables expected, let alone the expectation of an implementation plan.

When this failed, a small king's ransom would be paid to hire an outside consultant, resulting in a slow death by PowerPoint. The consultants often would talk to committee members with real knowledge of the issue and then repackage this information back to the unsuspecting administration with overwrought graphics and contrived data displays. Again, there would be no specific deliverables or legitimate implementation plan. Usually, by this time, the senior administrator in charge would leave and we would be told the plan was on hold until the administrator's replacement could "look at things with fresh eyes" and "put their stamp" on it.

The new VP would arrive (everyone seemed to be a VP or an Associate Dean) and a new committee formed…. followed by a consultant… and by then, it would be time for a new VP. Round and round and round, over and over and over again. This works just fine in the fantasy football league. When anyone would ask about an operational issue, the answer always was readily available: "We have formed a committee to look at this." Or "We recognize the importance and we have hired Buford and Thornton Enterprises to make recommendations." Or "We have asked Mel Waslooski, our new VP, to prioritize this when he arrives next month."

*Dear Leader X,*

*In general, there are many, many meetings (commonly in the middle of the day) that we are asked to attend, that displace clinical activity. Shouldn't someone be accountable for explicitly defining the goals and deliverables and for creating an actual work product that makes us better, enhances one of our missions, and /or addresses a clearly defined issue with an expectation of an actual action plan?*

*I have a great group in my section…do not want to indoctrinate this learned helplessness, malaise, and expectation that all problems are unsolvable. A few "wins" would really help.*

*Neil*

Perhaps needless to say, the overwhelming majority of service issues never improved. But in the insular world of fantasy football luxury boxes, no one usually knew, so who cared? Senior leadership had to rely on the physician leaders, who in the end, didn't really have reason enough to become mired in routine patient care issues. When issues from the real world bubbled up to the luxury boxes, the committee/consultant/new VP cycle would create the appearance of action. Core problems rarely were solved as senior leaders were not in a position to know and physician leaders often benefitted personally from choosing not to tell them.

The communication gap this generates with the rest of the physicians is bridged with messaging. The organization becomes functionally divided between those who message and those who are messaged. Managers are armed with "talking points" to communicate to care providers. I don't think senior leaders understand the damage this causes to morale and a sense of shared mission when misinformation is messaged to those who are in a position to know the truth. Many decisions that need to be made by a healthcare organization are not easy and some in the organization may disagree. But leadership should make principled decisions that we can be proud of, tell the truth and let the chips fall where they may. The assumption is that surgeons/physicians/nurses are incapable of understanding complexity and that misrepresentation and mischaracterization are preferable, as they suppress dissension. In reality, fear of honest communication and viewing the truth as optional undermines institutional culture and effectiveness.

*Dear Senior Leader X,*
*I know I am a pain in the ass, but I don't think folks in leadership realize how inadvertently divisive messaging/repackaging the facts is. Why not just tell the truth, explain the basis for decisions, accept that not everyone will agree and be accountable for it? I think most*

*folks just want to know that the process was honest and we did our best.*

*Neil*

As mentioned, I was the Division Chief of General Surgery at UVM (and Colorectal Surgery at UChicago), as well as co-Director of the Digestive Disease service line at both institutions. It is my nature to be irreverent and rely on humor when issues seem to be taking on more seriousness than they merit. When one of my professional friends would take on an administrative role, I would send them the glossary I created below to get them ready to interact with the luxury box culture. It can be like moving to a foreign country that speaks an entirely different language.

### *Messaging*

*Selecting and merging bits and pieces of information to form or influence the opinions and actions of the stakeholders. The message is typically designed to be incomplete, misleading or overtly deceptive. (For those of you without an advanced degree in healthcare policy or business, we no longer use the former term "lying" to describe this latter circumstance).*

### *Stakeholder*

*The group of people to whom leadership believes they need to message.*

### *Meeting of the stakeholders*

*An event arranged by leadership for one or more of the following purposes:*

1. *To create the appearance of input and participation.*

2. *To blur the line between activity and achievement.*

3. *To avoid making the difficult decisions required of those in a position of leadership.*

*NOTE: Hiring a consultant can typically achieve the same goals but at a greater cost.*

### *Transparent/Transparency*

*A descriptive phrase that is universally used by leaders to convince stakeholders that a process is legitimate despite the obvious appearance of impropriety. It is widely believed by administrators that this term has magical cleansing powers. A person using this phrase is believed to be absolved of any responsibility for the integrity of their actions. Further, the process or communication so described is stamped with the imprimatur of legitimacy, earnestness and collaborative spirit, irrespective of its merit or fidelity.*

Aspiring physician leaders quickly learn the relative value of messaging instead of telling the truth. They learn that rising stars typically absolve themselves of the pesky burden of caring for the sick and become fluent in euphemisms, business slogans and luxury box language. They generally divorce what they say from what they do. Leaders learn the rules of fantasy football and how to excel in a world where real issues and real patients tend to become irrelevant. Instead, they create the necessary paper trail and buffers that protect them and enable career advancement.

Complete isolation of physician leaders is somewhat less of an issue in surgery. Surgeons understand that they really need to have at least a few toes in the clinical pond to earn the credibility and respect of their peers. There are still plenty of honorable and admirable surgeon leaders who successfully thread this needle and live comfortably in both worlds. I must again reiterate that this is clearly institution-specific.

Another major change over the course of my career was the appearance of email. Although there is little questioning how much easier it has made communicating, there have been highly undesirable consequences. Ironically, at the top of this list is how much easier it has made communicating. Almost anyone can instantaneously forward a problem to hundreds of people in the organization instead of trying to solve it. There is an immediate ability to respond without thinking first.

The biggest time waster and morale killer of them all is the "reply to all" email. Problems just circulate in cyberspace for weeks and months on end without resolution. Countless people can appear to be working on an issue without actually doing anything.

## THE BREAKING OF THE SURGEONS

One easily may receive a 100 or more daily emails, the vast majority with information that is entirely useless or irrelevant to the recipient. Sending, receiving and forwarding emails can consume a whole day and become a full-time job for many.

Those who perform legitimate functions in the organization, like surgeons, need to find a spare minute here and there to scan the relentless email barrages and identify the occasional communication with meaningful content. Not only does it waste enormous amounts of time, it provides access to surgeons from everyone in the organization 24/7/365 for functional junk mail or mundane matters that could clearly wait. Like the electronic medical record (EMR), email destroys the barrier between work and one's personal/family life.

Email eliminates the need for people to see each other, talk with each other and relate to each other as people. It eliminates the kind of conversations that teach us how we can help each other do our jobs. Prior to email and the EMR, I knew just about every physician in the institution personally; we would have shared a cup of coffee, talked in person or on the phone many times and recognized each other by sight -- even if just for a simple hello in passing. Now, colleagues are merely electronic presences; one may walk by them in the halls every day and not know who they are.

Similarly, the EMR largely has been a workplace disaster and is repeatedly cited as a major factor in physician burnout. Studies have suggested that physicians spend perhaps two to four hours each day in subservience to the EMR. Again, this connects the surgeon to the workplace 24/7/365 and makes one's home and personal space constantly vulnerable to "attack" and wanton violation.

Email and the EMR have made it simple for administrators to instantaneously unload administrative tasks to those who provide patient care. Since the administrative structure is often siloed, requirements rain down on clinicians from all directions, often redundantly, and typically reflect a lack of understanding of how workflow occurs in the trenches. Most often, it is the clipboard nurses who are busy creating forms from their respective isolation booths, resulting in the care team filling out the same information over and over again.

The impersonal method of remote, electronic communication also inhibits the necessary familiarity and personal interactions between mid-level administrators and the healthcare delivery team, yet suffices to create an electronic paper trail to satisfy the appearance of "collaboration" in the fantasy football league. In reality, it creates a sense of learned helplessness and chronic lethargy among nurses and physicians who have no way of making the madness stop.

For example, every time the hospital attorneys added a new requirement for the surgical consent form (e.g. consent to have medical students in the OR, photograph the surgical specimen or take videos of the procedure), it would be added to the form below the previous signature slot. With each new addition to the form, there would be another requirement for patient and physician signatures, making the process more onerous and time-consuming as the piece of paper gets passed back and forth over and over again. This would have been easily addressed if additions were placed above the signature line on each updated consent form.

Dealing with administrative leadership was a tough issue for mid-level managers/administrators on our team who tried to act as a bridge between the two worlds. It never worried me that I might be relieved of my limited administrative roles. But for our section administrators, it was an entirely different story. They were really good people and I never wanted them to put their careers and opportunities for career advancement at risk. The last thing I wanted was for them to be viewed as troublemakers who undermined the performances of the fantasy football league or proved incapable of checking the appropriate box.

They were the ones who heard it from the nurses/physicians when they were told to implement uninformed, foolish processes. Often these section administrators were caught between a rock and a hard place. What do you do when you know something is wrong but your superiors are heavily invested in the status quo? What do you do when you know surgeons are rightfully aggrieved and the leaders who control your job security and career advancement opportunities are programmed not to hear it?

Much of the unnecessary bureaucratic work on the physician side is offloaded to housestaff. They are perceived as the low ones on the totem pole and dumping on them is usually the path of least resistance. Too often, their educational needs take a back seat to the needs of administrators and more senior physicians. When combined with the reflexive and continuous bombardment of pages housestaff receive from nursing and the laboratories, their well-being and ability to function effectively can be severely compromised.

Several years ago, a three-month audit at UChicago indicated that the junior resident on our acute care surgery service was paged an average of 70-80 times per 24 hours. How can one possibly provide thoughtful responses, take care of patients or learn in this setting? This is another consequence of the career pathway for advancement in nursing that takes nurse leaders away from patient care areas. Nursing leadership compensates for the lack of "boots on the ground" experienced leaders by normalizing nurses paging the resident for just about anything and everything. Unfortunately, this directive (implied or actual) undermines nurses' learning and initiative and can diminish perceptions of their critical role in patient care and outcomes.

Residents in training are also the dumping ground for almost any iterative task required by other parts of the healthcare system.

Disregarding the residents' educational needs undermines the claims academic medical centers make about commitment to their mission as educators. No one walks into the middle of a high school and pulls the students out of class every time a tray needs to be cleaned in the cafeteria. Teaching hospitals typically don't hesitate for a second with their learners.

It once was clear what various departments in a hospital did. For example, there was housekeeping and medical records. Now, there is environmental services (EVS) and Health Information Management (HIM). HIM has become particularly important in its more recent role of helping make a hospital's patients appear as sick as possible, leading to higher reimbursements. The appearance of caring for sicker patients also improves comparative risk-adjusted outcomes for institutional rankings. Making this spin function go has largely been offloaded to housestaff. HIM team members are trained to direct a seemingly endless onslaught of queries to any resident who may have encountered the patient until they get the desired maximum billing phrase into the EMR.

One night I was watching the news and heard the word "gaslighting" for the first time. Within days, I heard the word three more times and read it twice. I had no idea what it meant and was a bit embarrassed that a word that seemed to have become so common was foreign to me. I looked it up; it was a true revelation. This was EXACTLY how the upper layers of management controlled their interests, coated themselves with Teflon and kept inconvenient truths away from the organizational senior leadership. Bad news/trouble in the ranks was to be withheld by gaslighting the truth teller or at least thoroughly washing and sanitizing the facts so no one would look bad.

When PINOs were unable to contain an issue and it bubbled up, the first move was to act like it was some sort of exception. This was fascinating when it occurred at a leadership meeting that included not just PINOs but physicians who were practicing medicine and actually using the systems. These physicians would know that a particular policy or process unnecessarily made things difficult. The initial response by the responsible PINO was to hush things up and say that they would take the matter up "offline" or act surprised and "explain" how certain circumstances beyond anyone's control had caused an isolated incident. And the PINO would close by saying things were well on the way to being remedied thanks to their insightful leadership.

Experienced physicians understood the message: it was time to be quiet and don't spill the beans….especially if you wanted to have a future in the luxury boxes or didn't want to make a powerful enemy. But if one physician pushed back, others would feel comfortable speaking up; it was hard to see a colleague being gaslighted. When less experienced physicians would speak truth, a senior physician leader (e.g. Department Chair) would step in and calculate whether to participate in the gaslighting or thread the needle by promoting a well spun, watered down version of the concern while still supporting the PINO.

It's never fun to see someone thrown under the bus for speaking the truth and caring about what's right. Many times I would get a confused call from a bewildered junior colleague after a meeting, trying to understand what had just happened and why the issue raised was so obviously mischaracterized. Did the PINO or senior leader really think what they said was true? Why was everyone else so quiet while an acknowledged, serious problem that harmed patients or created rework for providers was being swept under the rug? Did we just agree that the earth was not really round?

Probably the most egregious offender at UChicago was a senior physician leader in another department. He spoke eloquently and knew all the right phrases/euphemisms to make activity sound like achievement, wallpapering over ineffectiveness. Even his description of the applicable activity was fake, let alone the claim of some sort of accomplishment. The explicit goal seemed to be that senior-most organizational leaders would believe something innovative (or at least legitimate) was happening, problems were being thoughtfully addressed, a sound strategy had been formulated and the implementation plan was rolling out. Since many other physician leaders were primarily focused on legacy issues or national/international acclaim (and not clinical/operational issues), he could flourish.

With the proliferation of Zoom rather than in-person meetings, it became possible to present different faces to different constituencies at the very same time. This senior physician leader could give different responses and present a different truth to different audiences almost simultaneously. For example, a surgeon might raise the concern that our transfer center could only get a very small fraction of patients who needed/wanted our help brought over to our institution. Transfers were a near-constant source of angst, as this leader well knew from his personal involvement.

When the issue was raised on the Zoom call, he might act surprised and ask with feigned concern for the name of a patient to whom this happened so he could "look into it," as if it were a one-off (gaslighting 101). In the "chat," multiple other physicians would indicate that they had the same issues. He might respond in the group chat out of site to senior leadership that he was grateful for all of the feedback and imply that he would vigorously pursue a solution. In a chat message directed only to an individual, he would talk about his frustrations with institutional "mediocrity" and how eager he was to sit down and talk personally about the acknowledged problem.

On many occasions, I reached out to this senior leader privately to discuss a thorny operational issue. He would often disparage the institution, apparently to seem sympathetic to the concern and offer to meet. I would express appreciation and indicate that I would gladly meet any time he was free. Almost invariably, I would never hear back, even after multiple attempts to reach out. He might then see me walking in the hall weeks later and would suddenly pull out his cell phone as if he just got an urgent text (concerned look and all) and try to avoid eye contact. Intentionally, I would walk up to him and say hello (yes, I admit it was fun). He would act surprised (like he hadn't seen me walking towards him) and perhaps tell me how he had been out of town, had some issues come up that kept him hopelessly busy, or the sun was in his eyes and try and make small talk. The meeting never would occur.

This is the prototype of a physician leader who can thrive in the fantasy football league rules and culture -- a disingenuous politician who doesn't seem to let the needs of patients or the care team interfere with personal ambition and seeks only to simulate the bi-directional communication that actually could create synergy and trust between senior leadership and physicians. To the Dean, CEO, or President, the message is all is just fine on the field; to the physicians in the trenches, you have a friend and advocate in me. It never seemed clear exactly where patients or truth fit in this narrative.

# Chapter 4:
# Melvin and the Tostitos

It always was disconcerting when a physician leader appeared indifferent to the needs of patients, such as those in need of transfer to our hospital -- a baby who needed specialty care, a patient in a local Emergency Department with an apparent complication of a surgery done at our institution or those whose outcome and life would be very different in a tertiary/quaternary care setting such as ours.

*Dear Senior Administrator X,*

*I still could not get a coherent story from the transfer center regarding the problem. We need to be accountable when our patients are in need of evaluation and care after surgery here.*

*Dr. Y has still not met with me -- I really need to have an opportunity to meet with senior leadership. We need to have an explicit understanding of the goals and rules so we don't do this dance every week. It is exhausting as the re-work and constant backtracking/cat and mouse game are intolerable and strain our relationship with our patients, referring docs and hospitals.*

*If we don't want to take transfers, let's acknowledge it.*

*Thanks*
*Neil*

## THE BREAKING OF THE SURGEONS

*Dear Manager Y,*

*I just hope for the sake of our patients that the culture in the transfer center changes, that folks are more thoughtful and consistent in what they do....and that leadership takes more of an interest in understanding the dysfunction, what is actually happening and the impact on our patients and their families.*

*I like the folks at the transfer center -- most are very nice. It is the policies and culture that are the problem.*

*Respectfully,*

*Neil*

Often, we would have patients who were receiving neoadjuvant therapy (radiation and/or chemotherapy) with us for six or nine months prior to planned major cancer surgery. Days before the surgery date, one might get copied on an email chain (reply to all, of course) indicating that our institution does not accept the patient's insurance for surgery and the operation could not proceed. After nearly a year of multidisciplinary planning, physician visits, radiologic studies and intensive treatment, the rug would be pulled out from beneath our patient and their family.

We knew and cared about the patient. We had worked hard optimizing their health status to make the operation as safe as possible. We knew and cared about the family. We had grown close and worked hard to gain their confidence and assured them we would do our very best for them. We had blocked off a full day in the operating room for a major operation with our team and arranged for other specialists to participate. The patient and their family had made the arrangements to have their support system available; family had taken time off from work and were flying in from out of town.

*Dear Senior Leader Z,*

*As leaders, we really need to make it clear to our staff and managers that the goal is to solve the patient's problem. Taking care of patients here (especially complex patients) is a constant uphill battle as the culture is so profoundly lethargic and ineffective. We need some accountability in the system as it harms people and consumes hours and hours of provider time (if you care enough to try and do the right thing).*

*Hope the enclosed list of individual cases might help.*

Thanks,

*Neil*

Now that the procedure was only days away, the system got around to checking the patient's insurance and pulled the plug by "reply to all" email. It felt horrible putting another human being through this -- but to the administration, the patient was just a name on a form and a holder of the "wrong" insurance. They had the "right" insurance for lab tests, x-rays, radiation and chemotherapy --

but not for surgery. It didn't even seem to make sense financially for the institution.

*Dear Manager Y,*

*Please escalate to senior leadership as surgery has been planned since March and his surgery was booked in June. We just cannot wait until August, the week of the planned surgery, to address these issues as our routine.*

*From my perspective, it is a horror show that we do this to patients so often (acknowledging that the insurance companies have a role in it, too). But from the institutional side, it must be evident/common sense that routinely canceling our cases the week they are planned results in unused OR time and loss of revenue....is anyone in charge???*

*NH*

Sometimes, the denial turned out to be a bureaucratic mistake, and after countless phone calls and engaging in a dizzying array of reply to all emails, this could be remedied. On other occasions, it was possible to escalate to a senior leader and get things back on track. It helped enormously if you were sufficiently senior for them to be willing to engage with you or at least respond to the inquiry. Otherwise, the junior surgeons had to enlist someone sufficiently senior, like their section chief, to get attention paid to the issue.

Something that really should be handled with a single phone call with a reasonable and responsible person, would turn into a chaotic morass of redundant and beside-the-point verbiage. It often seemed that this was the goal: make the system so onerous, insane and time-consuming that one would throw in the towel and stop advocating for what felt like basic decency. I always hoped I was wrong about that.

*Dear Manager X,*

*I appreciate your acknowledgment of how this issue impacts individual patients who rely on us. I fully acknowledge that these decisions/negotiations re in/out of network are difficult and may require tough decisions.*

*My concern is that we continue to approach this by sending ever-expansive reply to all emails (presumably hoping someone on the list will do something) instead of actually taking responsibility and managing the problem.*

*Why we would wait to act until days before a planned procedure is beyond me.*

*But let's focus on my patient. I had asked our section administrator to manage this issue this a.m., as the approach had continued to be emails that just go round and round. This man was referred with cancer associated with another chronic condition. I need to be forthright and upfront with him. We have acted irresponsibly by waiting until days before the surgery to address this. We should do this procedure. But I will respect a thoughtful and considered decision. I will not respect the continued neglect of this patient and a continued casual approach to his needs (or at least a disinterested approach devoid of accountability).*

*Please resolve this BY PHONE with Y* **TODAY** *and let me know what is decided.*

*Thank you*

*Neil Hyman*

Similar issues occurred in the setting of care continuity. For example, a patient might have an unavoidable change in their insurance in the middle of treatment while they were awaiting a second-stage operation. Or, they may have had an emergency procedure at UChicago and were then denied the reconstructive procedure needed to make them whole again.

For example, I had cared for a young woman who lived on Chicago's South side, who had come into the Emergency Department with an intra-abdominal abscess related to a localized diverticular (colon) perforation. A radiologic drain was placed and she was sent home with the tube in place to be optimized for surgery (colon resection). Of no surprise, we were informed that she could not have her diseased colon removed at our hospital. She called the clinic on several occasions to let us know she was draining stool from around the tube on to her abdominal wall. When I spoke with her, she tearfully explained that the odor from the drain was intolerable. She was sure she would lose her job as her coworkers could not tolerate the smell. Similarly, her kids were embarrassed to have her pick them up at school as their friends could smell it, too. She was devastated and humiliated.

*Dear Senior Leader X,*

*I need to escalate a situation regarding a patient with a diverticular abscess who has been admitted twice -- it's a young woman of color with two kids who has been draining stool around her drain for 2 months and we can't even get a response to our appeal of her continuity of care denial here.... it's exhausting and disconcerting that our physician "leaders" don't even have the integrity to identify themselves so we can have collegial discussions instead of bridge to nowhere reply to all emails.*

*This issue really does take up an average of ½ hour of my time every day just spinning my wheels.*

*Thanks*

*Neil*

This sort of scenario happened over and over again and caused considerable moral distress to our team, including our nurses and housestaff. Patients would keep coming back to our Emergency

Department and would have something temporizing done to enable them to be discharged. The only other option available to us was to do immediate urgent surgery, potentially involving greater risk and a colostomy that the patient might otherwise not really need.

The process at UChicago for out-of-network patients, where there were issues of "continuity of care" denials, consisted of a relatively perfunctory form that was reviewed by one of four or five physicians. You were not allowed to know which physician reviewed the form and you never knew when you would hear. This unnecessary uncertainty was awful for the patient, their family and the care team. We just wanted to make a sick person better and were stuck over and over again with telling this suffering person that we had no answer for them and could not say when we would.

Sometimes, we would ultimately get approval but other times, we would be denied -- no explanation provided and no opportunity to speak with whomever at UChicago had made the decision. We would appeal and wait indefinitely until the undisclosed physician issued their decision. I would highlight that even an insurance company allows peer-to-peer (physician-to-physician) conversations when care is denied. Why was it not possible for the Chief of Colon and Rectal Surgery/co-Director of the Digestive Diseases Center or ANY physician in this circumstance to have a collegial discussion with the UChicago physician making the decision, explain the circumstances and hear the basis for denial?

Was it really so terrible to ensure the treating surgeon that the administrative physician understood the applicable circumstances and potential consequences, considering they only had access to a very limited, standardized short form? Remarkably, it was not even thought necessary to have a surgeon as one of the physician adjudicators to decide surgical cases. There were two or three internists, a radiologist and a pediatrician. This approach really spoke volumes about how the institution viewed its obligation to patients and how it valued the surgeon's need to fulfill their professional oath.

*Dear Senior Leader Y,*

*This is just an awful situation that we raise over and over and over again.*

1. *I don't know why we wait until the week before to verify payment for a surgery booked a month in advance-we create these crises, respond with a relentless barrage of reply to all emails, and act as if we have no responsibility or accountability. How awful for the patient and their family who have entrusted us with their care (in this case for ~ a year).*

2. *Do not understand why the approval process for care continuity is secretive -- even the insurance company lets me speak to a peer. Here, we just file the form (sometimes over and over), waiting for some unnamed administrative physician leader to*

*evaluate. The patient calls us over and over and we cannot even know if the request is being considered/what the timespan will be for a response.*

*I had a patient a couple of months ago leaking stool out of a colocutaneous fistula who had two previous admissions here related to this. We filed at least three times and heard nothing for over a month; I tried to get someone (anyone) to help me figure out how to get a response -- her children would not let her pick them (and friends) up from school because she smelled... her co-workers complained and she expected to lose her job. I finally gave up and got her set up somewhere else, but wouldn't it have been better if I could have talked to someone? Even if they said "no," I could have gotten this taken care of elsewhere much earlier.*

*It really seems shameful and inexplicable.*

*Thanks*

*Neil*

In a Zoom meeting with the PINOs and other senior leaders, I again brought up this point. When the usual gaslighting response was given that this must be a one-off, other colleagues joined in. One of the hand surgeons explained how difficult it was for patients to be seen with a tendon injury and sent out without repair. These patients would be unable to work and support their families without the use of their hands. A trauma team member talked about the consequences for teenagers who were sent home with a colostomy after being shot and not allowed to be brought back for colostomy reversal.

It was hard to justify why we let young moms walk around with stool coming out of their belly, why we let workers with a family to support walk around with a hand they can't use and why we let teenagers in very challenging situations in their formative years of life navigate adolescence with a colostomy. The response of the senior-most operational leader nicely encapsulates everything I have been saying about messaging and the rules of the fantasy football league, "We don't want to disturb the healthcare ecosystem on the South side." The implication was that we were actually heroes and altruists…. who knew?

It is unfair to blame UChicago for the failings of our country's healthcare system, and there are safety net hospitals where presumably, people could receive care. But in many cases, care continuity is critical to a good outcome. And it's not like many patients from the South side could just scroll down their contact list and find another colorectal surgeon -- or had access to a primary care physician who could make a referral. We needed to help patients navigate the system and make realistic plans for them to get the care they need. In my experience, I'm not sure I ever saw this happen.

When email became the dominant method of communication, so much was lost because people no longer had the need to speak with their colleagues, especially those who work in other departments or other parts of the organization. People are no longer people; they are merely an electronic presence. Coworkers do not have conversations, do not really understand each other, do not accrue the respect and trust that results from personal contact and do not build the relationships that actually make things happen.

More ominously, suspicion and ill intent are allowed to fill this communication vacuum. Disrespect, demonization and a loss of a sense of a common mission become endemic, as does personal and professional isolation. As an old timer, I still would call and/or reach out to an individual when something meaningful was actually being addressed. Turns out that many administrators who worked at UChicago also had children, did not eat their young and took pride in their work. And they were commonly at least as frustrated with the dysfunction, disingenuous messaging and lack of achievement. A lot of really good people work there.

Just as the EMR would explode the ratio of activity to achievement for care delivery, email did the same for operational effectiveness. Both have been devastating for quality patient care, workplace satisfaction and the ability of healthcare organizations to actually get things done.

"Reply to all" emails are particularly onerous because they tend to create multiple, parallel lines of conversations that often conflict. It is seldom clear if any actual action is expected; just one misunderstanding anywhere in the chain leads to another hopeless trip into a rabbit hole. Yet reply to all emails have become normative because so little effort (e.g. forwarding an email/replying to all) is required to create activity, get your name dispersed to a wide audience and provide the façade of some sort of achievement. It is stunning the number of folks in modern healthcare whose job boils down to sending and receiving emails and they often don't like it any more than we do.

*Dear Manager X,*

*It's so inappropriate to send reply to all emails to lists of physicians asking "Someone" to complete a patient's death certificate. I have reviewed the 9 reply to all emails so far -- I will take responsibility and be the "Someone" you refer to in the email. I have directed this to Dr. Y in my section, who cared for this patient and will complete it.*

*NH*

Further, there is the constant waste of time sifting through mountains of electronic garbage so as not to miss the one relevant communication. For example, one might be copied on a reply to all email that Melvin in Accounting is being promoted. I've never met Melvin, but I am happy for him. The email announcement is sent across the organization; 388 recipients reply to all, congratulating him. Someone sends a reply to all email indicating that there will be a reception in the Accounting break room today to celebrate. I'm sure Melvin is a nice guy, but it turns out there are patients with colon cancer who need surgery today, so I will not attend. And since Accounting is in an off-site building and only a handful of folks know Melvin, I expect that very few of the other 13,000 employees included in these emails will attend the reception.

Thankfully, minutes later, I am also informed by organization-wide reply to all email that Edna is bringing Tostitos; this is followed by a reply to all email that Buford is bringing the dip. Rufus will be a bit late as he needs to stop by Employee Health to get his flu shot. Nice to hear that Morton has known Melvin since they worked together in Purchasing and remembers that he really likes potato chips. Six or seven reply to all emails later, all 13,000 employees no doubt are all relieved to learn that snacks are amply covered. There is also an email that the back-up generator for the loading dock will be tested today -- who knew that this also required all employees to read and reflect upon it? Thank goodness our administration is being so "transparent" and "reaching out."

There are physicians in leadership positions who clearly have a moral compass, did not consider care delivery to be a menial task for suckers and wanted to help. It's important to acknowledge them personally, as these attributes score them no points in the fantasy football league and do not get them a better seat in the luxury box.

They needed to know that the physicians on the field were noticing and were appreciative.

*Dear Leader X,*

*I am retiring end of next month. Leadership here has really been sorely lacking...largely smoke and mirrors and disingenuous performative orations. In obvious contrast, you are clearly very earnest and know the difference between activity and achievement. You are standing out high above everyone else.*

*Your genuine concern and dedication are clear. Most others have been unable to hide their narcissism. Just wanted you to know some of us notice and appreciate, as it makes us all better.*

*Neil*

# Chapter 5:
# Infinite and Free

It is not only physicians who are adversely impacted by the increasing sequestration of those who lead the organization from those who deliver care, make the sausage and generate the revenue that supports leaders in the luxury boxes. It almost feels like an emerging apartheid system with the "haves" in the luxury boxes and the "have nots" on the field. The income differences are staggering and increasing logarithmically. The evolutionary changes in nursing serve as a cautionary tale -- the nursing administrators and rank-and-file nurses barely know each other anymore. No wonder nursing unions (something I never imagined back in the day) seem to be gaining power. Nurses want to be valued and they care what happens to their patients.

The communication gap and experiential as well as physical separation of nursing administration (the NINOs -- Nurses In Name Only) from the nurses on the front line taking the daily hits has had devastating consequences as I described. Leadership seems unaware how tone-deaf and disingenuous their messaging sounds. It just can never make sense that there is ALWAYS plenty of money for massive pay raises for senior management, yet funds NEVER seem to be available to support the nurses, physicians and their teammates who care for patients.

Indeed, the pay gap between hospital senior leadership and nurses is expanding even faster than had been thought. A report from North Carolina "Hospital Executive Compensation: A Decade of Growing Wage Inequity Across Nonprofit Hospitals" noted that many hospital CEOs recently quadrupled their salaries in just a few years while nurses' pay largely stayed stagnant. According to its executive summary:

*"Nonprofit hospital executives have enriched themselves while fueling a crisis of health care affordability. North Carolina's nine largest hospital systems paid 'highly compensated' executives more than $1.75 billion from 2010 to 2021. Almost 20% of that hospital executive pay was captured by a small handful of hospital chief executive officers (CEO), who collectively took home $308.8 million over 12 years."*

As Dylan Scott noted in his February 2023 *VOX* article:

*"Hospital executives are seeing their compensation increase at even faster rates than previously calculated, even as many of them continue to fall short in providing charity care to their most marginalized patients. The pay disparity between hospitals' administrative staff and clinical staff is exploding: Some of the individual hospital CEOs covered in the study saw their salaries increase by more than 700 percent in just a few years, while doctors and nurses got a fraction of that salary increase, 15 to 20 percent, across an entire decade.*

## THE BREAKING OF THE SURGEONS

*Taken together, the study paints a picture of hospital executives enriching themselves at the expense of vulnerable patients and overworked staff."*

*Dear Senior Leader X,*

*I understand that nursing shortages and retention are indeed a national problem. However, I continue to think it would be helpful for the OR manager to visit the operating room every month or two so he was familiar with some of the issues and showed the staff that they were worth an occasional visit.*

*Neil*

And if leadership continues to treat physicians as interchangeable employees and fails to respect and value them, the physicians will be next. There is no amount of messaging or email barrages that can compensate for the need to feel valued, heard and treated fairly or serve as a substitute for the professional responsibility surgeons have and feel for their patients.

Although progressively diminishing, physicians may be the only "non-administrators" with any power left. Based on personal relationships and street credibility from working shoulder to shoulder at the bedside, our coworkers frequently turn to us for help being heard. They feel powerless to advocate for patients and remedy injustice or administrative unresponsiveness. Back in the day, nurses collaborated with surgeons as a matter of course, building individualized solutions for patients based on their shared goals. Nurses could approach one of their senior colleagues or the nurse leader, who also worked on the unit and had a shared experience -- and almost always could lean on their personal relationship with surgeons.

But now the system is fundamentally broken, the connections largely non-existent or severed and nurses often feel powerless to fix it. No one credible has a direct line to the luxury boxes and the rooms where it happens. And the process to communicate is incredibly tortuous, opaque and blocked by indifference or willful ignorance by those who are fundamentally committed to maintaining the status quo. Institutional leadership is now a self-serving oligarchy, largely inaccessible to the rank and file.

The system has not collapsed already because physicians and nurses have shown time and time again that they will do whatever it takes to help their patients. But times are changing, people only can put up with so much garbage and this house of cards will ultimately crumble without systematic change. As Dr. Danielle Ofri observed in her June 2019 *New York Times* Op-Ed, "The Business of Health Care Depends on Exploiting Doctors and Nurses: *"One resource seems infinite and free: the professionalism of caregivers."*

Referring to the challenges of caring for patients in the modern healthcare arena, she notes that *"quandaries are standard issue for doctors and nurses. Luckily, the response is usually standard issue as well: An overwhelming majority do the right thing for their patients, even at a high personal cost.*

*For most doctors and nurses, it is unthinkable to walk away without completing your work because dropping the ball could endanger your patients. I stop short of accusing the system of drawing up a premeditated business plan to manipulate medical professionalism into free labor. Rather, I see it as a result of administrative creep. One additional task after another is piled onto the clinical staff members, who can't and won't say no. Patients keep getting their medications and their surgeries, and their office visits. From an administrative perspective, all seems to be purring along just fine."*

My apologies if this sounds gratuitous, but I really do love and admire nurses. They work so hard, do so much good and put up with a lot of nonsense. I hate to see them disrespected or their good nature taken advantage of by clueless and thoughtless policies and directives. I feel the same way about the other members of our care team -- the medical assistants, front desk staff, etc. In so many cases, their association with our team and/or the institution is fundamental to their identity, dignity and sense of self.

By generating so many foolish, time-consuming tasks, by having all communication be one way (i.e., seldom inviting or valuing their expertise and experience) and by imposing broad-brush directives that make no sense in an individual setting, administration destroys the esprit de corps and employees become disengaged and feel disrespected. The good ones typically quit and those who have no problem with an "all activity and no achievement" culture stay. They just follow the rules, spin their wheels in the prescribed manner, keep their head down and collect their paycheck.

Dealing with tearful/frustrated nurse colleagues and advocating for loyal and committed support staff increasingly became a part of almost every day. There were constant false assurances and chronic systematic unresponsiveness to their needs and issues they raised. For the mid-level managers, "dealing" with these issues meant initiating a reply to all email extravaganza involving countless other mid-level managers. The most minor and straightforward personnel issue easily could take a year or more to address, let alone resolve. This was not because someone objected or there was pushback, but because "this is how we do it." Again, nice folks; horrid system.

*Dear Director Z,*

*Our patient access specialist quit because she was told she should mind her own business regarding patient access. Whenever she would identify patients with cancer who were spending weeks in reply to all purgatory waiting for someone to actually get them an appointment with a colorectal surgeon, she would offer to intervene, break the email chain, and get the patient in right away. She knows it is our sectional policy to offer all new cancer patients a visit within one week (irrespective of template or full schedules).*

*This is particularly ironic as you may recall that our surgical team had our service line bonus cut as we did not meet the metric for the percentage of cancer patients seen within 7 or 14 days of contact. What can we do differently other than be willing to add any cancer patient to our schedule at any time?*

*Neil*

And when we are so consistently unable to solve basic problems, we end up losing our most valued staff and end up with…well…what we end up with.

*Dear mid-level manager X,*

*I think it's really important regarding fairness and retention of key personnel that we get issues like this resolved in less than 6-8 months. I am not blaming anyone and understand that these issues can be associated with various complexities and nuances. But we also have to understand how frustrating it is for someone who has worked here for so long and is so committed/loyal to UCM to know that brand-new folks with less or no training and no experience are being hired at a much higher salary….then to have salt poured in the wound by having to teach these folks how to do the job and correct their mistakes……and not be able to get any explanation or timeline from their supervisor for when this will be addressed.*

*Thanks*

*Neil*

*Dear mid-level manager Y*

*Hi, when you have a moment in the days ahead, can you please stop over to my office (a few doors down) instead of continuing to email me and explain why this issue has not been resolved?*

*Hard to understand what "progressing" means, as this is what she has been told for the better part of a year.*

*Thanks*

*Neil*

As one of my colleagues explained to senior leaders, *"Position Control's constant and prolonged obstructions to clinical care is clearly the most objectionable issue that is frustrating our faculty. This entire process needs to be overhauled to one that HELPS us deliver care, not hinders it."* And I added, *"Sometimes the administrator needs to get off Zoom, leave the office, talk to/get to know the people who work here, and see things for themselves."*

## THE BREAKING OF THE SURGEONS

Dealing with basic, bread-and-butter issues for our team and support staff was a constant source of frustration. Certainly, most of my surgical colleagues cared for our support staff, who were so instrumental in enabling responsive care. But the system was so onerous, unresponsive and opaque that a sense of resignation and learned helplessness permeated the ranks. There just seemed to be nothing one could do to help care team members and coworkers be recognized and treated fairly. This even extended to basic issues like employee safety.

*Senior leaders X and Y,*

*I am really at wit's end regarding these folks. For the past 3-4 weeks, my administrator and I have sent well over 15-20 emails to managers we have been directed to, almost always with no response. I got bounced all over the place when I tried unsuccessfully to speak to someone by phone last week. The bottom line is that our physician assistant is a young woman who needs to come in some days quite early in the am (when it is dark) and/or leave quite late (again when it is dark) owing to the demands and nuances of our busy service.*

*She has expressed OVER AND OVER again (with progressive fear and angst) that she feels unsafe walking back and forth to the Drexel garage at these hours. As you might expect, the recent events on campus have only served to exacerbate these fears.*

## THE BREAKING OF THE SURGEONS

*We can perhaps have reasonable "supply and demand" discussions regarding parking access (I know these issues are not always easy). But the fact that the responsible leadership clearly does not take these concerns seriously enough to even respond to emails/calls/inquiries is very disconcerting; this really undermines and mocks the high-level messaging we keep getting about employees being "valued." It makes people want to leave.*

*In the end, I care about her. The casual and callous approach to her safety concerns really is unacceptable. I would greatly appreciate your assistance. Thanks very much in advance for your help.*

*Neil*

One of the most disabling euphemisms was a "team approach" to sometimes even the simplest of problems. Almost any issue would be forwarded to a vast array of "team" members so "everyone would be in the loop." There has to be some issue that just can be dealt with by the person who receives the initial inquiry. Clearly, many issues are best dealt with by a consistent individual rather than a team. Team is a nice word and a nice concept, but it has come to mean that nothing will be done and no one held responsible.

For example, patient complaints or concerns are usually very difficult and need to be handled individually with sensitivity. A major illness or operation is often a time of severe anxiety and vulnerability for a patient and their family. It is a time when mistakes are poorly tolerated and misunderstandings readily abound; forthright communication, empathy and kindness are crucial. The bureaucracy inherent in the "team" approach often requires a patient or their family to repeat their account to multiple, different representatives and typically sidesteps clarity with respect to who will respond and when.

This tends to reflect poorly on the surgeon, who only may learn about the issue when the "team" has created an unshakable sense of unresponsiveness to and stonewalling of the patient and their family. Surgeons, by their nature and training, are used to taking responsibility for their actions, including care of their patients and communication. Casually distributing a complaint to a broad array of institutional personnel can unfairly smear a surgeon's good name and reputation.

The complaint often represents a readily remediated misunderstanding. I always wanted to hear about these issues directly and right off, especially when they involved my junior colleagues. This was a time for mentorship and support rather than institutionalized shaming and often represented a teachable moment.

*Dear Manager X,*

*I don't believe that if I were a patient in this situation, I would be soothed/feel respected by form letters from multiple sources as the exclusive institutional response to my concern. I would prefer to have someone who was actually listening to me and helping me navigate the system. Even if that person was out sick today, I would prefer to get a callback tomorrow rather than being told to call the representative du jour.*

*I am always surprised by how liberal we are in sharing these personal letters with such an extensive list of people. It is humiliating when they involve my junior folks (like this one), and they don't hesitate to say so.*

*Thanks*

*Neil*

The changing culture and the relative openness of younger surgeons on the challenges of handling adversity have been refreshing. When I started, I thought that all surgeons were in total control of their emotions, especially after a bit of experience. I distinctly remember a conversation I had with a senior colleague after my first complication. I had operated on a delightful older woman with colon cancer and she returned to the hospital two months after surgery with a small bowel obstruction. I understood very well from training that this was a relatively frequent complication and occurred as a natural but undesirable consequence of the healing process. It was highly unlikely I had done anything wrong

## THE BREAKING OF THE SURGEONS

I came to see her that evening in the Emergency Department and spent the entire night wide awake, wondering if there was anything I could have done differently at surgery. I reviewed the operation over and over in my mind, even though I knew all about the idiosyncratic nature of adhesions and small bowel obstruction; they occurred in everyone else's patients too, and there was "nothing to see" here. By morning, I was annoyed with myself for my irrational oversensitivity. I ran into one of my more senior colleagues and admitted how "childish" I had been. I could quote all of the relevant studies and describe the pathophysiology of small bowel obstruction. But it still felt awful and that I had let down my patient -- even though she was as kind and as reassuring as one could be. She even had thanked me profusely for coming to see her in the evening!

I asked this senior colleague how long a surgeon needed to be in practice before these unwarranted feelings of guilt and self-questioning stopped occurring after a complication. He smiled his familiar little smile and answered, "never." It was a simple but profoundly enlightening answer and one that I never forgot. I recognized that the very moment these feelings go away, it's probably time to pursue another line of work. Although I certainly got much better at handling complications and other adverse outcomes, I never, ever, became dismissive of them.

This "second victim syndrome" is very real and can cause burnout, post-traumatic symptoms, depression or worse. But to be honest, much like burnout, generally I was unaware of the impact and extent of this phenomenon throughout much of my career. Ultimately, experience delivered me from the realm of the completely clueless. I got pretty good at identifying it in my junior colleagues (and myself) and recognizing when to step in.

# Chapter 6:
# Soap and Great Service

When I was at UVM, I was asked to co-lead an operational redesign effort in conjunction with an outside consultant. This experience introduced me to many aspects of the organization more broadly, with which I had basically no knowledge or experience but now needed to understand. My interviews with administrators were right out of the movie "Office Space" and its TPS reports.

I would sit down with someone who would tell me something like they were "Assistant Coordinator for Environmental Reconstruction and Integration." I would apologize and admit that I had no idea what that meant and asked if they would explain. They might then explain that they "oversee implementation and coordination of integrative strategy in the Vermont biopsychosocial milieu and ecosystem." Still baffled, I would ask if they had any function in enabling the hospital to act in a more environmentally friendly and sustainable manner. I would then be told that this was another department and they were focused on "human infrastructure."

After several similar demonstrations of futility understanding terms and positions I could not begin to fathom, I changed approaches. Someone would come in and tell me that they were the

"On-site Manager for Cross-Disciplinary Mission Communication and Services." I would ask the following questions:

1. Let's assume you have just arrived on campus. Where would you park?

2. Where is your office?

3. Let's assume you are in your office and have had your coffee; you make a phone call. Who might you call and what would you talk about?

4. Let's assume you are off the phone now. You are headed for a meeting. Who would be at the meeting and what might be the agenda items?

If I still couldn't figure out what they actually did, I would ask them to explain what the impact on the institution would be if they or their team were successful.

So, I was not really surprised when I came to UChicago and saw how dysfunctional things were. I was an Ambulatory Medical Director for the surgery clinics, so I had considerable interface with the outpatient settings as well as the hospital. The most basic operational systems and procedures were functionally unfit. There were numerous phone numbers for the same clinic (only some of which were in service) being distributed to prospective patients and referring physicians. Phones were not answered by someone who could help a patient or referring physician.

## THE BREAKING OF THE SURGEONS

Clinic schedules were pure chaos and access remained awful despite many open appointments. Patient records from outside physician offices often were requested five or six times by various people, yet still would not be available on the day of the patient's visit. As noted, the system for insurance verification was abysmal. Patients could not reach their provider. Appointments could not be coordinated, so a patient living far away may have had to come back to Chicago three times the same week to see physicians in three different specialties for the same problem.

These deficiencies and challenges had been acknowledged by just about everyone I spoke to, in and out of administration, when I was being recruited. UChicago really is a wonderful institution with a rich history. But folks knew that these inefficiencies, ineffectiveness and overall lethargic culture were just unsustainable in today's competitive world of healthcare delivery. Institutions that could provide reasonable service were eating our lunch year in and year out. What I didn't know is that operational improvements would continue to take a distant back seat to keeping senior leaders entrenched and comfortably secluded.

The electronic medical record (EMR) has been a nightmare for many physicians. The "efficiency" it created included the ability for administrative departments such as Health Information Management to seamlessly offload their work to physicians. The EMR readily generates vague or automated queries that flood the physician's inbox or reply to all email carousels, making simple documentation issues painful and full of angst for the physician. A list of medical record "deficiencies" that were not even current would be launched into cyberspace, creating confusion and boundless rework. No one seemed to care.

*Dear Mr. X,*

*I am respectfully sending this in the hope this is the last reply to all email in this barrage of reply to all emails (that includes at least two people who do not work here anymore).*

*As the Medical Director, I used to reach out to the individual surgeon verbally when there was a persistent deficiency -- it quickly became clear that the majority of incompletes were already addressed, as the list you guys send around is up to a week or more outdated by the time all of these emails are forwarded.*

*When you send these mass reply to all emails, it is unclear who you are asking action from. It's very nice that I get a series of emails wishing me a blessed day, but I would really prefer instead (or in addition) an action that takes care of the problem. Every time I have a "deficiency," it is because there is some EPIC glitch that prevents me from signing my note -- it can get pretty frustrating and time-consuming that the response is more reply to all emails rather than an offer of assistance to solve the problem.*

## THE BREAKING OF THE SURGEONS

*Here is my recommended workflow instead of reply to all email after reply to all email:*

1. *When there is a deficiency, just directly alert the provider.*

2. *If the problem is not remedied in, say, 72 hours, contact the applicable administrator.*

3. *The administrator touches base with the provider and solves the problem (e.g. gets EPIC support involved).*

4. *Escalate to the medical director if the problem is provider resistance.*

*We just need to try and work together to make this a more feasible/efficient place to provide care.*

*Thanks*

*Neil Hyman*

This was one of my favorites. For years in the operating room, perhaps half of the soap dispensers did not function properly and the surgeon may have had to walk around the operating suites from room to room to find one that worked so they could scrub for surgery. This issue remained unaddressed and unfixed through my last day of work.

However, I can report that after two years, the related toilet paper issue was resolved! When I would walk into the OR bathrooms made for one, often, there would be no toilet paper. Sorry to be graphic and crude, but everyone knew to go upstairs to the locker room depending on the need.... But for women especially, this was a real pain and it was clearly a bit embarrassing for them to keep complaining to their superiors about a lack of toilet paper. The charge nurse was wonderful and also had complained to OR management week after week after week -- but it continued to be beyond our institutional capacity to fix. Having these sorts of hygiene "challenges" in an operating room seemed crazy, considering the lengths and expenses we went through to reduce perioperative infection risks.

*Dear VP X,*

*Respectfully, this is not going to be solved with an ongoing barrage of emails. Here is my suggested solution:*

1. *Find out the name of the EVS person who cleans the OR.*
2. *Tell her/him to check the soap dispenser.*
3. *If it is empty, put more soap in.*
4. *Find out who is in charge of fixing broken soap dispensers.*
5. *If the soap dispenser is broken, have the EVS person report it to the person who fixes it.*

*We can use the same approach for toilet paper. This issue has been raised countless times over the years (I have raised it repeatedly and escalated). Hoping you will give my solution a try, as*

*I think it will work better than the reply to all emails...we have tried that approach many times already.*

*Thanks*

*Neil*

This general issue became even more irksome during the COVID crisis. There were signs all over the place about hand washing, providers were wearing space suits to care for patients, people were being sent home from work and patients were dying from COVID infection. Yet, similar to the OR, we just could not get the soap dispensers on the care units reliably refilled. I escalated over and over, including to our Infection Control leadership who indicated they were powerless on operational issues. Here is a representative dialogue with the administrator in charge, although I also escalated all the way to the top, often with pictures.

*Manager X,*

*Respectfully, I am really tired of dealing with this issue. This is the soap dispenser in front of room YYY, where my patient has been for a week -- the soap dispenser (as have a number of others on this floor) has been empty since last Friday. We have notified EVS, and the nurse manager and I have reviewed daily with his primary nurse. We are in the midst of a COVID epidemic and are working hard to reduce our surgical infection rates. Every time I raise this, there is a flurry/barrage of reply to all emails, and ultimately, the one dispenser gets refilled one time -- this is why once a year, I include senior leadership. I really do not know why keeping these dispensers filled seems beyond our operational capabilities and appears to be such a low priority.*

*Let me again reiterate my annual recommendation-there are housekeepers on every floor; they should carry soap on their carts; when the flag is up and the dispenser is empty, they should refill. Rather than just sending reply to all emails in response to this issue, I would recommend that periodically, you or one of your staff make rounds on the floors to see if this is being done.*

*Thanks*

*Neil Hyman*

His response:

*Dr Hyman, I wanted to let you know the dispensers outside of room YYY have now been filled. I'm sorry that these have remained empty for several days without being filled.*

*I do want to let you know we are trialing dispensers that we get alerts daily notifying us which dispensers are nearing empty and also notifying us regarding batteries that are almost dead. This has the potential, if the software works correctly, to help us stay ahead of empty and dying dispensers.*

*We will continue to work to ensure great service to you and your team. Please don't hesitate to reach out to me directly if there's ever anything I can do.*

*Manager X*

My response:

*Manager X,*

*Respectfully, this email is just silly and seems insincere after several years of inaction, reaching out to you directly and letting you know what you can do to fix the problem.*

*Here are the facts:*

*Soap is necessary to clean your hands. Empty soap dispensers mean the healthcare team cannot wash their hands, which puts patients at increased risk for infection, promotes the spread of nosocomial infection throughout the wards, and drives up hospital costs. Patients rely on us to advocate for them and protect them from bad outcomes. Over and over and over, I report that the soap dispensers are empty for days on end... year after year. Every so often I escalate yet again to senior leadership. It is clear that there is no system in place (at least a reliable one) to manage this and the folks who take the calls for environmental services typically do not know who their managers are or how to address the problem. Hard to imagine this needs a high-tech solution or pilot project.*

*I have received some version of this email quite a number of times now...and several times from you.*

*My suggestion is to mean what you say and actually manage the situation and not just send patronizing emails. This is "great service?"*

*We should be able to have soap in the soap dispensers -- not a complex issue. I do have a suggestion to solve the problem instead of emails. Every day, have the housekeeper assigned to clean the room check the soap dispenser, which is just outside the door. When it is empty, have them use the soap container on their cart to refill. Expect this will solve the problem.*

*Neil*

This conversation, in one or more forms, continued for years without resolution. It seemed silly or maybe even abusive to send this all the way up to the top of the food chain repeatedly. But emails about unprecedented times, transparency or how excited we are were not going to get it done. With all of the endemic institutional gaslighting of physicians who raised issues like this, you had to reflect on whether this really was a hill to die on. How many issues could you escalate and still have an opportunity to have an impact? Finally, I started routinely sending pictures of bathrooms with no toilet paper, empty soap dispensers outside patient rooms, and filthy public bathrooms in patient care areas...some were quite graphic and I had to remember to delete them before I got home to avoid being kicked out of the house or arrested...

*Dr Hyman,*

*Thank you for your constant vigilance and for taking the time to report your findings. These issues were escalated by senior leader Y to the senior most leaders of our EVS service provider.*

*Please know that we are in the midst of a major redesign of our EVS/PT services, including all standard work processes. Our goal is to reset the department on the track to providing high-quality services and to do so in a highly reliable manner.*

*Please know that there are daily discussions on these issues and that a path to improvement is on the way.*

*We share your frustration and sense of duty to make things better for our patients.*

*Sincerely VP X*

*Dear Senior Leader X,*

*Earlier this week, I sent VP X a note with pictures about the vulgar condition of the bathrooms in patient care areas --bathroom after bathroom that is filthy, in some cases with blood on the walls, toilet paper all over the floor (in some cases "used") and other bathrooms without available paper towels or toilet paper.*

*Over and over and over again, I have contacted EVS that the soap dispensers in the operating room, outside the patient rooms and inside the rooms are not being refilled. I have escalated to the head of EVS on several occasions.*

*I inevitably get a patronizing response about the desire for "great service." The response cannot always be bloated emails about unprecedented times, transparency, and messaging. This is not a complicated issue. When the soap dispensers are empty, we need to put more soap in them.*

*I spoke with the nurses today as my patient in room XXX has had an empty soap dispenser since last Saturday. It has been reported many times by nursing but still not attended to. When I spoke with the nurses, they highlighted the number of soap dispensers that are empty despite repeated reporting. They took me around the corner to show me signs that have apparently been up for days now, alerting housekeeping and asking them to refill. I have sent pictures of this multiple times to management.*

*We just cannot continue to approach this by adding filters to reports and email chains. EVS needs to be accountable for doing their job. It is issues like this that alienate the physicians and staff. Thanks*

## THE BREAKING OF THE SURGEONS

*Neil*

I was always curious about what was going through the minds of the senior leaders in these situations. I knew that if I was in their situation, my instinct would be, "there is no way this can be true." The applicable manager always sent emails that everything would be fixed. Because I worked in the hospital and could see things for myself, I could readily see this did not happen. I am sure if I was in the C-suite, I would think that there must be some misunderstanding for such a simple problem and the issue has to be isolated. Without first-hand knowledge, I might be more inclined to trust the gaslighting responses of the applicable manager. It's just too hard to believe that replacing toilet paper is beyond our managerial capabilities. This is why it's so important that senior leaders take a stroll out of the luxury boxes periodically and have a look around.

*Senior leader X.*

*There are so many key operational aspects of our institution that are only managed virtually and this is one of them -- with euphemisms and messaging but limited or no actual action, even when it is as simple as this one. It is really unsettling to those of us involved in patient care and leads directly to the major issues we have with physician engagement.*

*Neil*

## Chapter 7:
## Don't Say Yes

One of the most gratifying aspects of being a surgeon is working together with peers outside of your own institution to improve care in your specialty. Most often, this occurred organically, but overarching regional problems could be addressed by more formal organizations such as the local chapter of the American College of Surgeons (ACS). When I worked in Vermont, we put together a statewide collaborative to improve cancer care and reduce complications. There are so many similar examples across the country and it's really a tribute to the commitment and professionalism of surgeons. Despite the potential for distrust and parochial institutional issues, the vast majority of surgeons put their patients first.

When colleagues would ask me about living and working in Vermont, I would often say, "it's great living so close to the U.S. and you can get in without a passport...." I'm not sure who I heard that from. The quality of life is excellent and the people are wonderful. I also enjoyed and appreciated the egalitarian approach to life and healthcare. UVM was the only large hospital in Vermont (although Dartmouth was just across the border in New Hampshire and much closer for people who lived in southern Vermont). In a small state like Vermont, you feel very connected as you are aware that the choices you make about resource utilization can impact your neighbors in a very tangible way.

Hospitals might have 25 or 50 beds and two surgeons. I had great respect and admiration for these surgeons. They were invaluable and indispensable to their communities and worked tirelessly on their behalf. They were very capable but usually did not have the complementary support structure or facilities to care for the most complex patients. I was the first colorectal surgeon in Vermont and there were four by the time I left. Like colleagues in other specialties like cardiothoracic surgery and transplant, we knew we HAD to accept all transfers as no one else in the state may be able to deliver the care for specific specialty problems. The institution was accommodating and we somehow managed to get the patient transferred in, even when there were "no beds" available.

Taking appropriate transfers is critical from so many perspectives. In rural settings, the larger institution may be the only one that can deliver the service to a patient. Further, this provides critical support to the communities with one or two general surgeons; they simply cannot easily see patients in the office, perform elective surgery, cover consults in the Emergency Department and attend to the minute-by-minute needs of a critically ill patient 24/7/365. These surgeons are human and need to be able to take some vacation time and attend milestone family events.

In addition, every surgeon has complications or things that do not turn out as hoped. This is a time when that surgeon needs collegial support, a kind word from another surgeon and not be hassled by the referral center with unreasonable requests and a "just say no" approach. I would explain over and over again to senior administrators how critical a strategic issue this is. If you treat the referring doctor respectfully and right, you will have a friend (and referring doc) for life. And it's just the right thing to do.

When I arrived at UChicago, it quickly became clear that the transfer center was a disaster for us. It never improved because no one seemed to want it to. I would not characterize the approach as "just say no" but more like "don't say yes." In the Chicago area, there are many centers capable of providing just about any kind of specialized care. My practice was largely IBD, reoperative surgery (e.g., for complications, postoperative fistulas) and recurrent rectal cancer.

When I would get a call from a referring provider with a patient in trouble, I would request a transfer (or the call would come into the transfer center, who would page me). Since the hospital was typically full (and insurance had to be checked first), it was uncommon that they could proceed with the transfer right off. I would call to check repeatedly and get one vague, noncommittal answer after another. I would hope to be able to see and assess the patient before going home at night.

After a series of nonproductive calls, the transfer center shift would change and we would start all over…commonly day after day. It felt horrible when a valued colleague would call to tell me the patient was still at their hospital and they were understandably worried about the impact of continued delays and the associated uncertainty. I would escalate to senior leaders and explain how difficult it was for the transferring physician to have to "sit on" a very sick patient (perhaps with their condition worsening), especially if this was related to a postoperative complication. Most institutions and providers just learned not to call us.

Senior leaders emphasize the goal of increasing volumes. But I don't think they understood how clueless this sounds to a surgeon when the institution prevented patients who wanted/needed our care from coming. Perhaps ~1/3 of colorectal procedures relate to acute problems -- the patients who are most likely in need of transfer to us. It is like refusing to allow ambulances to come to the hospital and wondering why the Trauma volumes are not increasing. Most patients who are shot, stabbed or in a car crash do not walk in off the street.

And then, as if to rub salt in the wound, we would get emailed about a strategy for "outreach" -- the goal being to try and convince these physicians, whose patients we were not accepting when they needed us most, to partner with us and send us their referral cases. A key component to the outreach strategy would have been to replace magical thinking and these oblivious policies with a respectful and accommodating approach.

*Dear Outreach Leader X,*

*Many thanks for asking for more details on what we discussed earlier. When I got here ~ 8 years ago, I spent a fair bit of time going out to communities to meet our referring docs (generally GI groups). Although they usually held the physicians in high regard, there was an incredible amount of animosity towards UCM with a perception of arrogance and disrespect. This largely came from two areas:*

1. *From their office staff:*

    *Requesting records over and over again for the same patient and telling them their patient could not be seen without records, even though they had already sent us several copies. I got a LOT of dirty looks and nasty comments from the office staff when they saw my UCM name badge, making it very clear to me that they did not like it when their docs made referrals to UCM. I think we have made improvements in this realm. However, it is important to understand that chaos/operational ineffectiveness can often be misconstrued as arrogance or even malice.*

2. *They do not get reports back from our visit or updates on care provided -- no consult notes, no operative reports, etc. Again, they perceive this as arrogance/disinterest when it really*

*reflects our operational inability to get records to them. We do not have a current address on many physicians and when there is more than one Dr Jones/Smith in Chicagoland, we usually had no clue which one is the referring doc. I often get my clinic notes sent to Dr. Smith, the ophthalmologist, rather than Dr Smith, the gastroenterologist. We just can't have an "anyone named Smith will do" approach.*

*To me, this is so simple; we just need the front desk to ask patients on check-in (and/or the scheduler who makes the appointment) to record who the patient would like records sent to. While they are at the front desk/on the phone with us, we can verify the doc's address, as the patients usually know this.*

*I can give you many examples of physicians who still have their original UCM contact information in our directory from when they did their training here decades ago rather than their present office address. There is one instance of a referring gastroenterologist I interact with frequently who has been trying to get his address updated since ~1992.*

*It's very disconcerting and provides an impression of arrogance and/or incompetence.*

*Thanks*

*NH*

## THE BREAKING OF THE SURGEONS

Like most major centers, we were trying to grow our footprint by acquiring hospitals, although quite belatedly. There was a remarkable lack of strategic clarity in many decisions, including acquiring a hospital where it seemed like few patients had insurance UChicago Medicine accepted. As we targeted new areas for referrals (outreach), our administration believed it should be built on talking points and messaging and even emailed instructions detailing how we should talk to our colleagues.

*Hi outreach leader Y,*

*I respect your work on this, but really do not think that messaging/talking points and explaining how "excited" we are to partner is the key to authentic and sincere communication with these physicians. We are all used to this sort of language from our administrative colleagues and know what it is; likely it will be perceived as insulting or worse.*

*I do not think that giving our docs a list of local physicians to call and going over the talking points (explaining how excited we are, how we are on message, how everything is harmonized and socialized) will be well received. Rather, I would respectfully submit that setting up meetings with key groups and a respected/trusted UCM colleague(s) who they interact with clinically based on specialty is the way to go.*

*Thanks*
*Neil*

COVID actually offered a glimmer of hope from the operational standpoint. These were trying times in so many ways. There was still the onslaught of reply to all emails from all of the administrators who worked from home. I had hoped that maybe COVID would cause them to reflect on whether performing their job by sending, receiving and forwarding reply to all emails really represented achievement -- and think about what physicians and nurses actually do all day -- no luck there. The number of staff working from home blasting the clinicians with a nonstop stream of emails became increasingly brutal and made me wonder if they were aware that the healthcare organizations' primary function is delivering healthcare to patients.

But there were also many very real and novel problems to be solved, such as protective equipment, appropriate OR use, clinical staff protection, visitation policies and virtual visits to name a few. I thought UChicago did a great job with this -- and hoped (in vain, as it turned out) that this could be a wake-up call.

*Dear Senior Leader Y,*

*It's just so disappointing. When we had COVID, we showed that we could respond to a crisis in real-time, not hire a consultant, not immerse ourselves in months of committee meetings with no agendas, not feign interest thru a relentless barrage of congratulatory emails or management thru messaging. We were just able to order the masks... set up COVID testing and move staff to cover COVID units. I am sad to see things going back to the old ways. It is worth striving for operational effectiveness and partnership in the real world instead of the virtual world, where the issues only appear to be addressed.*

*Thanks*

*Neil*

COVID also was a time to reflect on the workforce, as consideration needed to be given to who might be furloughed if things became nonviable economically.

*Dear Senior Leader X,*

*From 1975-2010, the number of physicians grew ~150%- around the same as the U.S. population; administrators grew by 3200%. Do we really need 32 administrators for every one we needed a couple of decades ago? There is so much vague thinking around what we need these people for. Maybe we should have an indefinite administrative freeze until we can assess exactly what this massive proliferating army of people is really doing. I do not mean this as a cheap shot or overbroad generalization. I just encounter so many people whose activity seems to be generating busy work for others.*

*Senior administrative salaries have almost doubled in the last 10 years; this is ~10 times more than the growth rate of physicians despite half the time required for education. Again, not meant as a cheap shot, but just don't know why that is and don't think it's healthy. Last data I have seen is that we are now at ~30% of healthcare expenditures on administration.*

*Thanks for considering,*

*Neil*

Again, I appreciated my time at UChicago and have so much respect for my colleagues and the institution's traditions. I derived so much joy from "my guys," what they were able to achieve and how deeply committed they were both to patient care and the academic mission. After COVID, I stopped agreeing to be part of things that were a complete waste of time, the things that were all about activity with no prospects for achievement. My time (and gratification) was focused on patient care, medical education/mentoring, career building for my team and supporting their efforts. They are truly a talented and committed group.

*Hi Guys,*

*Just wanted you to know that I have resigned from my position as co-Director of the Digestive Diseases Service line. There is no "back story" or angst; it is just that I am at the stage of my career where I do not want to participate in things that are not meaningful and impactful. I have not found this role to be either. I will continue to support our programs enthusiastically and hope to continue to be a reliable and supportive colleague.*

*Many thanks, and happy to chat. This is not a "take your marbles and go home" thing -- just do not want to continue in this capacity.*

*Thanks*

*Neil*

And thereafter, when administrative folks would ask for my participation in a committee looking at the same issue for the umpteenth time, but again given no authority or linkage to someone who might do something:

*Dear Manager X,*

*Thank you for reaching out and happy to support you/this. I do have one specific ask. I do NOT want to spend hours on Zoom calls introducing and re-introducing people, having everyone compliment everyone else, practice using their administrative vocabulary-building words, chant the word "transparency" and point out that they are "on message." I want to be sure that you are authorized to make a change and that there is a specific deliverable -- not just a slew of aimless meetings.*

## THE BREAKING OF THE SURGEONS

*I believe this to be an extraordinarily simple problem to solve and think it should take one 10-minute meeting. If the group is empowered to do something, I will happily participate.*

*Neil*

The inclusion of this and other emails, accumulated over nine years, may provide the impression that a large percentage of UChicago administrators were inept. Again, this is not why I included the emails and the correspondences typically represent the late stages of dialogues that went on aimlessly for months and more commonly years. Rather, the management structure was dysfunctional and the system detached from reality. I did find several senior leaders lacking in specific and important ways and maybe one or two overtly repugnant. It is disappointing to see leaders with talent, intelligence and the opportunity to do so much good instead use their position only for personal glorification and advancement (e.g., trophy trolling).

Quite often, junior administrators who were frustrated by their inability to get things done would reach out. Many times, I had never met them before. One emailed me after a meeting to express her frustration about systemic ineffectiveness.

*Dear Z,*

*Thank you very much.*

*You are clearly a terrific person. The problem is the profound disconnect between our administrative team and the folks in the trenches with "boots on the ground."*

*It is truly amazing how many folks create Zoom calls or meetings involving scores of us when there is no real agenda and no deliverables-the meeting consists of congratulating everyone, re-introducing everyone, "messaging" and trying to use the word transparency as often as possible, almost always out of context. The meetings are often scheduled during the day when physicians are caring for patients.*

*I am very sorry you feel the way you do and have a world of respect for you.*
*Thank you*

*Neil*

Finally, a letter to our new hospital President when he arrived. He was clearly a nice guy and I found him sincere. He expressed interest in improving our rating in *U.S. News and World Report* rankings. I had just resigned my "title" as co-Director of the Digestive Disease Service line. No one seemed to have the first idea of what the service line's purpose was, although it must have sounded like a good idea to have one based on what it said in administrative trade journals.

I continued to ask the senior most leaders exactly what the deliverables were, and no one could answer. My co-Director was a dear friend, a deeply committed clinician and a world-class academician. We had many ideas but no mechanism to have them vetted, let alone considered for implementation. For two years, our talented young administrator sat frustrated in his office with essentially nothing to do. I was nearing the end of my career and had no desire for a ceremonial position like this. I knew that having a title like this, where nothing was expected, would be very appealing to specific colleagues seeking luxury box accommodations.

*Dear President X,*

*Just wanted to personally thank you for coming last evening and for your thoughtful/candid remarks. I have spent over 20 years in a physician-leader role in academic medicine. I have always enjoyed the collaborative relationship with my administrative colleagues. In earlier years, I had been used to one of three sorts of responses:*

1. *That sounds like a good idea; put together a strategy/business/operational plan and we will review.*
2. *That sounds like a good idea, but we cannot afford it -- or now is not the time as this is really not a strategic priority.*
3. *That does not sound like a good idea.*

*All of these would work just fine for me. It has been many years since I have heard one of these types of responses. It felt good to have a sincere conversation.*

*At the level of leaders beneath you, the goal is to maintain the status quo and avoid engagement. It takes three common forms:*

1. *Just don't respond.*
2. *Forward the email to someone else.*
3. *When 1 or 2 will not suffice, create the appearance of some form of activity -- this could include:*
    A. *A committee with no charge and no expectation of deliverables.*
    B. *Bring in a consultant even if a very simple operational issue.*
    C. *Create yet another titled position and explain that the person needs to get their feet wet and have time to "put together their team."*

*I think your initiative re: USNWR is a classic example. It is clear to me (and most physicians) that this is now the coin of the realm reputationally. I offered to personally "scrub" the data on the colorectal cases to assess accuracy and work as part of a team to see what could be done to improve. I reached out to the senior person in charge over and over and could never get a response until a silly meeting was set up many months later with a lower-level person. She was very nice but does not have a medical background and really did not understand the issues. It was of no surprise to me that we did NOT rise in the ranking; it turns out that if all you do is message but do absolutely nothing else, the ranking does not get better.*

*I had respectfully resigned from my role as co-Director of the Digestive Disease Service line because there was absolutely no "there" there. Quarterly, I would get an email from the senior administrator in charge, essentially asking me if I could send over slides from one of our sectional projects (we do a lot of quality and access stuff in our section) so it could be presented to senior leadership as a Digestive Disease initiative -- implying to the Dean that we were actually doing some sort of work as a service line. It all seems to be about how best to game the system.*

*Many thanks and really do appreciate you.*

*Neil*

## Chapter 8:
## Burnout

I must be delusional about what surgical residency was really like 40 years ago. I suspect that nostalgia for the days of the giants distorts recall of the actual events and feelings that existed at that time. Somehow, just about all my memories are joyful or at least positive. But I know that there is no way this can be entirely representative of the relentless sleep deprivation, chaos and cyclical adrenaline highs and lows that we all experienced.

In fact, now that I am older and perhaps a bit wiser (although floor probably pretty low…), I have no doubt that many of my brothers and sisters in arms must have suffered mightily -- and it would have HAD to have been in silence. Conventional doctrine emphasized the distinction between those who were strong enough to maintain peak performance despite long hours, chronic stress and ongoing physical exhaustion -- from those who were not.

Surgical training was designed to ensure that those with the right stuff, who could bear this responsibility, had been toughened up and molded -- and those who could not would be weeded out. Patients were to be protected from those who could not be counted on in crunch time. It just never came up that any surgery resident could have depression or suffer from burnout.

## THE BREAKING OF THE SURGEONS

In fact, I don't think the concept or even the word burnout was in use -- certainly not in the world of surgery. I am utterly embarrassed to admit that I was 15 years into my career before I was even aware that there were any surgeons who did not love being a surgeon. How regrettably wrong I was. Looking back, I cannot decide if I had blinders on or have the emotional intelligence of a tin can.

My awakening to the problem of burnout happened rather arbitrarily. For better or worse, I was an early advocate of the concept of work-hour restrictions. I did not believe in a particular number of hours or rigid rules, only the sentiment that our residents did not need to go through what we went through to be well-trained and "join the club." There were aspects of training that just felt like hazing.

There are far more two-physician/two-professional relationships and it no longer seems reasonable (if it ever was) to ask a spouse/partner to put their aspirations and personal needs on the back burner for at least 5-10 years. I wondered what kind of role model would want their trainees to first meet their child at kindergarten graduation. I believed that our educational system was inefficient and there were major opportunities for improvement.

The work-hour restrictions question seemed to be framed as how could we possibly move our busload of parts (educational, experiential, historical) into a minivan instead of asking if we could easily get rid of some of the antiquated relics on the old bus, like the rusted Studebaker parts. Was it really necessary for all of the residents and medical students to wait at the nurses' station from 4:00 until 9:00 p.m. for the Chief Resident to finish operating before making evening rounds?

Even as faculty, I used to make rounds seven days a week for many years because I felt like I knew my patients best. But was that really necessary? Am I saying that my colleagues could not make rounds on my patients and give me a call if there was an issue? It was common we would all see each other at the nurses' station on Sunday mornings. Is this really "commitment" or is it just plain stupidity?

Anyway, I was serving as Secretary of the New England Surgical Society and was asked to give a talk on the concept of attending work-hour restrictions as part of a more general work-hour restrictions panel. It felt like I could be about to establish myself as the most despised surgeon in New England -- the kind of politically correct, namby-pamby surgeon who was coddling trainees and ruining the profession. I did some reading to prepare for my presentation and it was then that I first encountered the emerging literature on burnout. After the panel, I was asked to write an editorial for the *Archives of Surgery* in 2007 (now *JAMA Surgery)*, reprinted below with permission. I remembered that my email would be shared with the editorial and expected a nasty electronic whipping from the house of surgery. Boy, was I in for a surprise…

*"The personal relationship between physician and patient has long been the cornerstone of medical practice. The bond that is created between a patient and his or her surgeon is often forged in times of crisis (e.g., cancer or catastrophic illness), leading to a particularly powerful and special covenant. Because problems such as the development of a tumor, hemorrhage, or bowel perforation cannot be scheduled in an orderly manner during standardized hours, general surgery has never lent itself readily to a predictable work environment. A deep sense of duty and commitment to our patients, especially during critical times, makes the concept of work hour restrictions, or shift work, seem wholly unacceptable.*

*However, surgeons are human beings, parents, spouses, friends, and neighbors, too. Adequate rest and time for personal fulfillment are critical for individual well-being, especially in the challenging and sometimes contentious environment in which surgeons practice. Patients are not well served by an exhausted surgeon who is physically and/or emotionally burned out. These are the kinds of concerns that have led to work-hour restrictions for our residents.*

*Although there are conflicting data regarding the actual effects of the resident work hour restrictions, the concerns and criticisms expressed appear to be well founded. There are more handoffs; continuity of care has been disrupted, potentially leading to a diminished sense of professionalism and a shift worker mentality. Winslow reported that 70% of general surgeons perceived that care was worse, and 100% perceived that resident training was inferior after the work-hour restrictions took effect. Residents appear to know patients less well. Concerns exist about coverage, quality of patient care, and resident sense of responsibility and preparedness. Is this really a model we should follow? Further, these restrictions have had a significant effect on surgical faculty. Coverdill reported lower expectations of residents, less time for teaching, more work, more stress, and decreased satisfaction as work was shifted from residents to faculty.*

*However, it would be inappropriate to simply dismiss or denigrate all of the concerns that led to the work-hour restrictions. Although surgeons may consider themselves immune to human physiology, there is little questioning of the effects of sleep deprivation on performance. Wakefulness for 24 hours, a status well known to most surgeons, has been shown to be roughly equivalent to a blood alcohol level of 0.1%, the legal limit for driving an automobile. Cognitive function is clearly impaired. With regard to technical performance, surgeons awake all night have been found to make 20% more errors and take 14% longer to complete tasks on a laparoscopic simulator. Sleep deprivation is also dangerous to us personally. The risk of accident or injury, use of alcohol, weight change, conflicts with coworkers, percutaneous sticks, and falling asleep while driving have all been associated with extended work hours.*

*We must also acknowledge that young surgeons may have different demands and perhaps different values. At our institution, Gargiulo reported that concerns about lifestyle were by far the most important deterrent to a career in surgery among medical students. Surgeons increasingly must balance the career needs of their spouses and the demands of child-rearing while trying to keep up with the frantic pace of modern healthcare delivery. This must be accomplished in the setting of an increasingly cynical and demanding public, a hostile malpractice environment, and shrinking reimbursement. In a study from Washington University, general surgeons worked a mean (SD) of 73.8 (14.1) hours per week. Only 44% have at least one day per week that is free of clinical duties. Up to 95% of these surgeons are paged overnight at least once weekly, with a mean of 13.6 calls. Further, 73% return to work from home at least one time during the week. This all amounts to a recipe for burnout. In fact, evidence does exist to support this concern. In a study of American surgeons using the Maslach Burnout Inventory, 32% showed high levels of emotional exhaustion. Thirteen percent showed high levels of depersonalization, indicating that the surgeon viewed patients as inanimate objects and developed cynical feelings toward them. Burnout was more common among younger surgeons.*

# THE BREAKING OF THE SURGEONS

*Houston, we have a problem! We cannot continue to ignore the realities of modern practice if we are to attract the best and brightest medical students and allow surgeons in practice to flourish and enjoy the unique rewards of a career in surgery that most of us cherish. We are not superhuman and somehow immune to the effects of sleep deprivation. Do we really want our trainees to be absentee spouses and parents? Maybe we can learn something from our junior colleagues. On the other hand, we must avoid the rigid restrictions of the 80-hour work week that have compromised care and threaten to inculcate our trainees with a shift worker mentality instead of a professional work ethic.*

*We need to take a long, hard look at the way we work and consider the effect on our patients, ourselves, and the future of general surgery. Indeed, the threats of an unfavorable workplace environment on surgeons have been well documented and acknowledged by key surgical leaders. Perhaps surgeons on call at night in busy hospitals should routinely have the next day off. New paradigms of care, such as the surgical hospitalist model, need to be considered and evaluated with an open mind. We should demand that hospitals provide the necessary support personnel to complete the mind-numbing iterative paperwork that continues to proliferate in our healthcare system. Certainly, much of what we spend our time doing could be safely offloaded to other hospital workers without compromising patient care. The relentless proliferation of bureaucratic requirements that are imposed by third parties under the euphemistic banner of quality improvement needs to be vigorously combatted when the requirements do not improve the safety or outcomes of our patients. This "Dilbertization" of quality of care is a growing threat to our integrity and sense of professionalism. It is one thing to spend extra hours at work saving a patient's life or providing comfort and security; checking boxes and completing forms to satisfy meaningless directives is another matter altogether. We need to change or at least adapt to our new work environment; after all, who will be there to care for us when we retire?"*

*Neil H. Hyman, M.D.*

It's remarkable how understated and dated this seems now, all these years later. Several of my colleagues made kind and generous comments, but they were my friends. Instead of the blistering array of "you are Judas" letters I expected after this was published, I got maybe two dozen emails like the one below from a surgeon out West. Instead, I felt like the poster child for Master of the Oblivious.

*"I LOVED your article on Attending Work Hour Restrictions. I also love the (not so bold) statement, 'There is little questioning of the effects of sleep deprivation on performance.'*

*How many articles have been written to study this very question? How many times must we tell everybody that we are NOT supermen? We must sleep, rest, 'down time,' etc…*

# THE BREAKING OF THE SURGEONS

*By the way, do you know how many surgeons suffer from clinical depression but do not seek treatment for FEAR of medical board intervention or stigma? I dare say MOST of us do…but isn't it interesting that a doctor can be told, 'You are not safe to practice medicine because you're depressed.' But, if we seek treatment, 'You are not safe because you are depressed and are now medicated.'*

**I hate this job."**

*XXX M.D. FACS*

So much has since been written about burnout and there is no need to summarize all of that here. However, the incidence of burnout continues to grow with each new assessment and is being reported in astounding numbers in virtually every surgical specialty around the world. I was particularly bothered by the incidence in six general surgery training programs in North Carolina reported by Williford in *JAMA Surgery* in 2018 -- 75% of residents met the criteria for burnout, 39% met the criteria for depression and 12% of residents had suicidal ideation in the last two weeks.

How can we sit quietly while our trainees are at-risk and have almost no power to do anything about it? It is data like this and my personal interactions over many years with so many of these incredible residents and young surgeons that pushed me to share the reflections in this book.

## THE BREAKING OF THE SURGEONS

I am no spiritual guru or master of insight. Similar sentiments have been expressed by other senior surgeons in various disciplines, as in the following excerpted remarks from a 2023 publication by Daniel J. Waters, D.O., a retiring osteopathic surgeon:

*"For all the wonderful experiences that come with caring for patients, working with trusted colleagues, and just plain making a difference, there are a host of nagging injuries, the result of the sometimes brutal emotional collisions and concussions that we rarely talk about or refuse to acknowledge.*

*Perfect outcomes are always out of our reach, and treatment failures, missed diagnoses, and complications, not to mention the litigation that can ensue, are omnipresent threats. Some physicians are shielded by their arrogance, their avarice, or their ignorance – but I believe this is a very small group. The rest of us suffer the slings and arrows with barely a whimper and just keep moving ahead.*

*But these days, there are way more slings and much sharper arrows. And the fortress that used to be our office or the hospital has been breached by ruthless C-suite executives, more of which we seem to see every year. And places to find shelter or protection are rapidly disappearing. It started with pagers, progressed to portable phones and then to cell phones and iPhones. The IT monster that is the EHR and 24/7/365 online access to every nook and cranny of the* medical-industrial complex has stripped away the once-sacrosanct comforts of home and travel.

'They can always hurt you more,' a character in the book The House of God says. Now it's more like, 'They can always track you down.' We can work – work! – any hour of the day or night from almost any corner of the world where there's a WiFi hotspot or a cellular tower. And, more and more, it seems that's exactly what we're expected to do. What was once the unthinkable has somehow become the norm.

There is, in my mind, a fundamental difference between hanging in and hanging on. And that difference is, well, different for each of us. For me, it was the escalating daily battle with clueless and sometimes malevolent administrators, meddling middle managers, bumbling bureaucrats, and some of my physician colleagues who were more than willing to do their bidding that did me in.

I freely admit it: These people wore me down. If I were a football QB, I'd say I was getting sacked on every other play, and targeting was definitely not a personal foul. And I loved what I did. I loved playing the game. But in hindsight, I realize first I was sent to the medical tent, and then to the locker room, and then into the stands – and just in time, I'm convinced now.

We all, regardless of our specialty, take our share of hits over the course of our careers. Sometimes, we are, as the TV announcers like to say, slow to get up. But get up we do and shake it off, maybe *rub a little dirt on it. So, take a hard look at why you're still in the game. More importantly, take a hard look at the toll the game is taking on you – on your family, your health, your happiness, and your mental well-being."*

Like many other issues in healthcare that impact surgeons, most senior leaders generally have paid only gratuitous lip service to burnout. A number of cosmetic and/or disingenuous initiatives have been instituted. But this is not an issue that will be solved by the once-a-year free cup of coffee on National Doctors' Day. The increasing physical and professional separation of administrators and physicians will turn out to be very costly as we have seen with nursing. Being clueless about the factors that impact physicians' quality of life and ability to do their work makes it almost impossible for leadership to understand and solve problems. Relying on physician leaders (PINOs) for advice and counsel when they do not use the system and/or do not have an earnest or legitimate connection with the rank and file, results in the ineffective air ball strategies that predominate.

A few surgeon leaders have stood up and tried to move beyond the superficial rhetoric. But there really needs to be MUCH more urgency and willingness to stand up for the surgical community, especially for our residents and young surgeons. The vast majority of surgeons remain so committed to their patients and the profession that they just continue to put up with whatever it takes -- more hours, more bureaucratic requirements, more garbage and more disrespect. This can only continue for so long until the house of surgery comes down like a house of cards. Surgical leaders have got to stop focusing so narrowly on their own career advancement and cutting deals with those who create this environment. The focus must be on leading (rather than managing), promoting professional values and standing for something besides a budget.

I have tried to provide specific examples of how administrative bloat can make advocating for patients and staff a chronic, time-consuming irritant. And as opposed to administrators, a surgeon does not just go home at a certain hour. The surgeon must stay until all patient needs are properly addressed. The foolish forms, mandatory in-services, email barrages and hours of making unrequited love to the EMR are all extra.

No one hires more surgeons just to complete iterative work. In contrast, more work on the administrative side (whether legitimate or illusory) means more administrative hires and more mouths for the surgeons to feed. As noted earlier, 32 times more mouths to feed over recent decades. You would think healthcare institutions would place more of an emphasis on providing healthcare instead of growing bureaucracy.

Rather than the annual free cup of coffee or expanding the boilerplate messages of staff appreciation to include Arbor Day and Flag Day, there are a number of meaningful changes that would reduce burnout and make physicians/nurses far more satisfied with their jobs and more connected to their institution. Many would cost little or nothing.

For many in healthcare, the EMR may be the ultimate profanity. Perhaps no single factor has so adversely impacted healthcare delivery, professional satisfaction and physician effectiveness than the EMR. Having said that, it is not the EMR in concept that is to blame.

EMR acquisition and implementation was a monumental expense and a real budget buster for healthcare entities. Key decisions were understandably left to the senior administrators. Costs to implement EMRs for even small practices were in the hundreds of thousands of dollars and tens of millions for larger entities. Costs needed to be recovered, especially when it became clear that the EMR made physicians far less productive instead of increasing productivity as promised. In response, the EMR was re-designed and used primarily as a billing tool and a way for hospitals to provide the illusion of far more comprehensive care than was actually being provided -- so they could bill for it.

Much has been written about the impact of EMR on burnout. Physicians spend an average of 4.5 hours per day using/coping/battling with the EMR and it's reported that physicians now spend two hours dealing with the EMR for every hour of patient care they deliver. Obviously, this is not what any physician wants to do or what their patient wants them to do. But "optimal" use and EMR gamesmanship drive revenues -- and undermine basic ethics and professionalism.

Think of what we have trained and are training our next generation of surgeons to do. I think back to when I was in college and took Philosophy 101; my roommate had it the semester before. Say I asked, "Hey Bob, can I have that term paper you wrote last semester on Socrates' *Apology*?" If I erased his name, wrote my name instead and turned it in, it was called plagiarism. You might expect to be expelled. Now, it's called EMR and considered optimal practice.

We have normalized physicians copying and pasting the previous note from another provider and then representing it as their own, usually with a minimal addition. A physician is consulted for a skin tag that they inspect. With a few clicks, they can generate an 11-page note "documenting" 20 years' worth of X-rays they have never seen, reviews of organ systems they never asked about and extensive exams they have never performed. Finding something/anything meaningful, unique or sometimes even true in the EMR is a time-consuming scavenger hunt.

Large amounts of imprecise or overtly erroneous information are carried over from note to note and become the operational reality. Often, these medical "facts" are presented to or electronically accessed by remote physicians who make decisions based on billing-driven misinformation. Any responsible surgeon knows that they need to do the key parts of the exam and review pertinent history directly with the patient. But in some specialties, the EMR has provided the facade of comprehensive care when, in fact, the patient was barely touched. Rest assured they were amply and generously billed.

## Chapter 9:
# JOMO

Surgeons come to understand that their career success and livelihood are largely built upon reputation. So, when negative patient comments or complications are carelessly paraded around the institution's email circuit, there can be shame and feelings of abandonment. Don't get me wrong; accountability is a bedrock of surgical practice. Complications must be reviewed diligently to ensure patient safety is relentlessly pursued and optimized. But there is a right way, a decent way and a fair way to do this.

*To: Patient Relations*

*Subject: Patient Feedback*

*Hello, my name is HW. I am a patient under Dr. Y. I was admitted to the hospital for colon surgery this past Friday. I was told at the time of surgery that they would put me on a liquid diet right away. This was not done, and I tried for several hours to get answers from my care team. The nurses on my floor were very helpful, but nobody showed up until well after dinner. By this point, the cafeteria was closed, and I had to wait for food until the next morning.*

*I also had concerns about my pain management and frustrations waiting to be discharged. Needless to say, this level of inattentiveness makes me want to change my GI doc rather than risk being admitted to this hospital again.*

*If you need additional information, feel free to email me.*

Sincerely,

HW


The Patient and Family Insights Department (that really is their name) then started one reply to all email blast to our Clinic Manager, another to my Physician Assistant and a separate one that ultimately included me. Each one was copied to the entire "Insights" department and no responsibility was assigned. The familiar institutional approach is to send something into cyberspace to as many people as possible and hope someone does something. If not, there is a paper trail showing you forwarded the email and did your job. The patient gets an unsigned email with generic, patronizing platitudes about how important their issue is.

Ultimately, our Physician Assistant forwarded one of the email "conversations" to me to make it stop. I responded:

*Hi all,*

*I have dealt with this on our end. Let's not forward emails indiscriminately to an expansive circle of folks. It is unbecoming and unprofessional and does not protect either the patient's privacy or the nurses'/physicians' dignity.*

*We also will not be sending patronizing, unsigned notes to the patient but will actually try and do the right thing. I have spoken with Dr. Y and a personal conversation with his patient has been set up.*

*Thanks*

*Neil*

Patient complaints are usually well-founded but often result from misunderstandings that may not even be known by their surgeon. The phrase for the process of response is "service recovery." Most surgeons are eager (or at least willing) to have the opportunity to discuss troubling issues with their patients, explain things and reestablish trust if necessary. I could never get our senior leaders to understand this.

*Dear Senior Administrator Y,*

*This is what I meant when I was speaking with you. It seems so inappropriate to deal with each and every patient complaint with an ever-widening set of reply to all emails. I am not a lawyer, but this does not seem to be compliant with the spirit of HIPAA. More importantly, the utter carelessness and unprofessional nature of the process really upsets my guys (especially the younger physicians). Notice the letter to the patient is not even signed by anyone—if I were the patient, I would think I was being patronized by a cable company type response.*

*Really wish you guys would consider a different process. I do not understand why one person can't simply send these to me or my administrator. We care and would want to make it right. This approach adds all kinds of unnecessary and hurtful aspects.*

*Thanks*

*Neil*

At UChicago, we had a well-intended institute led by highly respected physicians that aimed to foster the doctor-patient relationship. They graciously agreed to sponsor a session on burnout.

*Dear Drs. X and Y,*

*What a wonderful program and so nice to hear from the physicians who participated -- rejuvenating and inspirational for all of us.*

*As you know, burnout is a growing scourge in our profession. I am well aware that this is a tricky issue to navigate, as many initiatives believed to make good business sense are in direct conflict with the doctor-patient relationship. Some degree of tension with senior leadership would seem inevitable. But I think the allowable space for the institute and its mission grows smaller and more limited by the day in an environment where business values dominate and physicians' values are marginalized.*

*Examples would be using Relative Value Units (RVUs) as the basis of compensation. We may lecture about empathy and spending time with our patients. But we are paid based on throughput and the physician who spends time consoling patients, has family meetings or calls their patients will likely find themselves "rewarded" with a pay cut. Physicians are so used to excelling and being high achievers; sending them monthly reports, perhaps indicating they are "performing" at a low percentile, is likely something they are not used to....and, in many cases, not something they can even control. In surgery, they may relate to a lack of OR access or the inability to have patients transferred here for care. They can't operate without an operating room, a hospital bed and support staff.*

*Of course, some of our physician leaders are great docs. But many are clearly NOT role models and do not demonstrate respect for the doctor-patient relationship. They are typically chosen based on their business mindset, willingness to look the other way and/or political savvy. Unfortunately, some are anything but respectful of patient care. We are messaged by our leaders with talking points created by the marketing/communication staff. The communication is generally superfluous and seems intended to enhance their standing among their peer administrators.*

## THE BREAKING OF THE SURGEONS

*I could not have more respect for the two of you. Further, I really do understand that this is a tough issue. But I am getting to the end of my career. I just hate to see such an enormous percentage of my junior colleagues feeling devalued and disenfranchised and the doctor-patient relationship viewed as a quaint relic from an earlier time.*

*Thanks*

*Neil*

For surgeons, the most obvious stressor might seem to be the operating room. However, doing the operation was often the easiest part of the process. Rather, it was getting the case scheduled or moving things along in the OR, so patients would not have to wait in the lobby with uncertainty and anxiety for hours -- and the surgical team could get home at a reasonable time. I enjoyed the anesthesiologists at both places I worked and really valued the warm ties I had with so many OR nurses. They were skilled, committed and a joy to work with.

But the inescapable fact is that only the surgeon has to stay until his/her cases are done and the other two groups of the OR team (anesthesiology/nursing) are generally working a shift. This creates an inevitable tension as OR inefficiencies in scheduling, access and performance preferentially impact the surgeon and patient. Surgeons alone are assessed by their individual metrics such as the number/complexity of cases and surgeons often feel isolated and alone in accountability for group performance. Whatever equipment issues, emergencies or operational/administrative failures lead to delays, it's the surgeon and patient who wait.

As a senior surgeon, you generally have the respect of staff, are better able to handle the nuances of disruptions such as emergencies and tend to have fewer unscheduled surgeries. The frustrations my young guys experienced in getting add-on cases done and emergencies taken care of in a timely manner were formidable. There were few things I hated more than seeing one of my junior colleagues sitting in the lounge for hours on end waiting for the OR to let them get started with a case, knowing that the surgery could have been done long ago if things were more efficient or someone in OR administration was managing attentively. Another night of a surgeon not seeing their little ones before bedtime -- this should matter and be a priority for the OR administration. But it isn't even on the administrative radar screen.

*Leader Y,*

*Here is yet another set of examples from yesterday where my guys had issues (details sent separately). I have to highlight how helpful nurse leader X has been in situations like this when she is made aware. It has made a huge difference both logistically and in surgeon morale.*

*But this approach has GOT to permeate the OR more globally as she cannot single-handedly change the culture. The charge nurse has GOT to have some idea of what is going on in the OR and be willing to leave the front desk to find out. They may see a room empty for hours and hours on end, and at no point does it cause them to investigate what is going on...while a patient waits anxiously in the pre-op hold and another has their surgery cancelled. And the surgeon has to be away from their family and miss seeing their children before they go to bed because no one in leadership is interested.*

*Somehow, the needs of patients and the personal well-being of surgeons (especially the young ones) have GOT to matter.*

*Neil*

There are so many other examples of things that make a surgeon's life more difficult that could readily be addressed if only senior leadership was aware and thought it mattered. But you can't fix what you don't see, what you don't know and what you don't understand. The PINOs and other physician leaders who interact with senior leaders have too often failed to inform and advocate because this does not advance their careers and isn't easily framed in the language of the luxury box. There is not always a direct budget impact to show, no business plan to review, no cost opportunity and nothing is being "socialized."

As noted earlier, some euphemisms like "shared responsibility" and a "team approach" often signify the death knell for problem resolution. This frequently means that there will be a group of folks who sit around simulating work and get nothing accomplished because nothing is expected and there is no pathway for implementation even when there is intent.

For example, I was often informed by the "team" that a peer-to-peer phone call was needed with an insurance company to obtain authorization for one of my patient's operations. Although a small number of these calls were understandable, most issues seemed straightforward as I did very little discretionary surgery. For example, a patient with colon cancer needs their tumor removed. I would ask our team (nice folks, by the way) what the problem was and always would get a response something like: "you know how these insurance companies are."

Then I would go through the hassle of waiting on hold, providing all kinds of bureaucratic data and then trying to find a time when I could manage to speak to the authorizing insurance doc. Time after time after time, I would be told that the insurance company had been asking for medical records from our administrative staff or were waiting for a diagnosis to be provided and had received no response to repeated inquiries. Rarely was there an actual issue to resolve. Rather, it was just customary to unload this on the physician rather than investigate what was needed.

## THE BREAKING OF THE SURGEONS

Despite the frustrations expressed about the operational practices of modern healthcare, almost none actually pissed me off -- this one did.

*Dear Manager X,*

*There is a big issue and a little issue with our approval process. There seems to be no clue that providers are here to treat patients -- not to attend meetings, respond to emails and do the administrative work of the people who get paid to do this work.*

*You said that because fax numbers change and providing medical records can be a challenge, you think it is appropriate to have physicians take time away from patient care and make these calls to be the preferred workflow? Your folks need to at least consider doing their job and helping solve problems.*

*Here are a couple of things I would highlight:*

1. *A peer-to-peer requires the physician to call and set it up -- this can include up to 30 minutes of hold time.*
2. *Then there is the actual call that needs to be scheduled the following day -- this is also extremely disruptive.*
3. *When I made this particular call, the insurance company physician indicated that multiple attempts were made to get records. Why do we choose to request a peer-to-peer instead of just sending the records and verifying?*

> 4. *Each time this has happened, I have responded personally to the UChicago person who sent me the request for peer-to-peer and told them it was once again a failure to receive records and not a denial and that the admission or surgery was approved. Not once have I received a follow-up call or email that explains what happened on our end; only another bogus peer-to-peer request for the next patient...lather, rinse, repeat.*

*Neil*

As a senior surgeon, I had access to plenty of support staff and had the experience to know how to minimize these sorts of disruptions. But the impact on junior surgeons and our residents was far worse. They are the ones who most need the support as they are at the highest risk for burnout. Almost always, their needs were ignored, trivialized and minimized. They did not have a seat at the table in the room where it happens and there was, for some, a sense that learning how to manage being "dumped on" is just part of "growing up" as a surgeon. Perhaps most importantly, young surgeons are not the ones who grant promotions, make appointments to senior leadership, hand out trophies or keys to the luxury boxes. So, they routinely get the short end of the stick.

I have some empathy for senior leadership relative to making decisions about which insurance to accept. Personally, I just wanted to take care of everyone and let the economic chips fall where they may; no doubt this at least partially explains why I would have been an awful CEO. The issues surrounding the patchwork of coverage, partial coverage and no coverage that defines the U.S. healthcare system make these issues complex. This is another area where it's easy just to throw stink bombs from the cheap seats. There is a lot of careful analysis and tough negotiations that go on in support of these decisions.

However, the impact these issues have on surgeon burnout is often overlooked. As opposed to the category of patient that healthcare system leaders need to consider (e.g., the patient with various private insurance coverages, Medicare, Medicaid or no insurance), the surgeon is confronted with a real patient with a name, a family and a very real disease that may be quite serious and potentially life-threatening. And we want to help; that's what surgeons do. Not being permitted to continue taking care of a patient, especially when it is someone you have come to know well and have cared for before, feels awful. The trust established with the patient and their family and the intimate knowledge a surgeon has of their condition is discarded, creating a sense of professional and moral emptiness.

*Look guys, we have been treating this man and directing his care since June of last year. I/we have been in touch with him and his son many times over that time interval. The plan has been for surgery all along. Again, this plan has been explicitly documented for 8 months* now. He has a very complex situation that cannot be cared for in his local community. We have known this for 8 months.

I totally understand that we do not make policies for insurance companies that we do not direct healthcare policy...and that negotiations between UChicago and insurers are not an easy issue. But we need to figure out a way to avoid this last-minute drama. Imagine that you are this man or his family, and UChicago has told you for 8 months that we would provide your care and do your surgery. His docs back home told him that this would provide him the best chance to be cured of his cancer. And then, at the last minute, we pull the rug out from under him.

We have to care more and be more mindful of the patients, families and referring docs who rely on us. I am certainly not the only one who can do this operation, but it is clearly not a procedure that can be done safely in his community. He would require a major academic center. The surgery is time-sensitive and would doubt that he could get plugged in elsewhere at the 11th hour and get the care he needs in a timely fashion. We deny the care based on administrative failure and leave it to the physician to explain it to his/her patient.

We really need to be better.

Neil Hyman

## THE BREAKING OF THE SURGEONS

At both UVM and UChicago, we had outstanding and deeply committed residency program directors. They did their level best to advocate for the residents but generally had few cards to play. Their ability to impact change relied heavily on the energized support from the Chair, who largely controlled their prospects for career advancement. I really appreciated the program directors' dilemma and commitment and hated to see residents getting dumped on just because they had such a limited voice.

*Dear Program Director Y,*

*Education Day is clearly one of my favorite work days of the year as it reminds us all how incredible our training program is and what a great program director you are; congrats, as the program makes us all very proud and is a tribute to your leadership and commitment.*

*I did notice the concerns the residents pointed out regarding the volume of nonphysician work that is required of them, and not sure where this stands relative to our peer institutions. But I do share that concern, as you know. I recently met with senior leader X, who was sharing plans to offload a lot of our coding initiatives onto our residents. He made the argument that this is actually a "good learning opportunity." I strongly disagree on a number of grounds and told him so. I think we need to watch this carefully, as the messaging around why these iterative tasks should be assigned to our residents really strains credibility.*

*Thanks*

*Neil*

Many of the mismanaged or unmanaged processes were dangerous in addition to being burnout promoters. Remarkably, our lab folks did not have access to identify which physician ordered a test, so they often had no way of knowing who to call to inform of abnormal lab tests or that a specimen was inadequate. They really only could call the Admitting Surgeon of record, even though that surgeon rarely had ordered the test (for example, it was ordered by the ICU team, a resident or a consultant) and may no longer be involved with the patient. Usually, they would not get a response to the page and start paging on-call surgeons who had no knowledge of the patient or the test ordered.

*Hi Manager Z,*

*Got paged from the micro lab again last night about a patient of mine in the hospital that a sputum sample was inadequate. No big deal, but she is in the ICU, and obviously, I did not order the test; also unclear why the tech could not just notify the nurse in the ICU that another sample was needed. So, at 2:45 a.m., I had to call in and notify the ICU nurse to collect another sample. I waited 15 minutes on hold for the operator and then again for the nurse to pick up. I also got called earlier in the evening about an outpatient sample issue on one of my colleagues' patients and on another sample for a patient I do not know.*

*Over the past 8-9 years, I have gotten well over 100 pages like this on hospitalized patients (usually waking me up in the middle of the night) as the person paging told me they had no training or understanding of who to call when there are issues with specimens (or abnormal labs). They are unaware of how to find out who ordered a test or aware that we have residents in the house…usually, they express surprise that I have called back because it is so seldom that anyone does. They just perceive the need to check the box and document that they tried to notify someone. This is dangerous and a real nuisance.*

*Over the past 8-9 years, I have had many discussions with lab directors but the issue never gets addressed. Can you see if there is someone at a senior level who I could address this with and who would actually consider trying to fix?*

*Thanks*

*Neil*

I had many conversations with lab techs, radiology staff and nurses in the wee hours and felt their pain as well -- they were just trying to do their job and didn't know who to call. The simple explanation was that lab staff did not have access to the EMR. All they had was the "requesting" physician's name, which was a default to the attending surgeon of record. They had no directory of physician office numbers for outpatients. This was never addressed, so the beeper could and often would go off night after night and weekend after weekend, potentially even when you were on a family vacation.

I asked several colleagues about this and they correctly pointed out that our residents had our phone numbers and always knew how to reach us when there was a legitimate issue. So, they either shut their beeper off or didn't answer these pages. Indeed, when I would discuss this in the middle of the night with the lab staff, they were always surprised someone answered the page. They just needed to document the attempt. I always worried that something important would slip through the cracks. Hard to fathom that something this easy to fix with such potential for disaster was just not considered important enough to remedy. Undoubtedly, I had more than 20 meetings or communications about this during my time there. Thankfully, I am one of those folks who always can fall back to sleep immediately.

*Dear Leader Y,*

*Hi and thanks for meeting with me. I have been emphasizing repeatedly how dangerous it is that our lab folks do not know how to find out who to relay critical lab values to, as they do not have EPIC access. I am routinely paged (often in the middle of the night) with handling issues/need for an order/wrong tube or lab results on patients I do not have primary responsibility for or may not even be involved with.*

*This happened three times last week alone. Have met with the lab directors (who seem to change every few months) and even sent them copies of the pages with patient ID, medical record numbers and time of page.*

*This issue has been escalated to many clinical leaders many times and not addressed; it should be straight forward -- informing the team of critical lab values, missing orders or mishandled specimens can be a critical safety issue.*

*Efforts to fix communication gaps or signs of legitimate interest across the organization for issues that put our patients at risk would be great. Thank you in advance for any efforts that can foster this culture.*

*Thanks*

*Neil Hyman*

Another time suck is the various mandatory training modules that continue to proliferate. The concept seems to be that if we make physicians and nurses spend their time viewing these PowerPoint or "interactive" third-grade level presentations, we can say that we are sensitized and that the organization takes an issue seriously. This might help with litigation or a public relations challenge someday, as we now can claim that everyone has been "trained."

Let's say that the institution wants to show it seeks to prevent work place intimidation. A "mandatory" is added and required of the entire staff. Maybe the surgeon gets up early on Saturday morning before his/her kids to complete the two-hour program.

Scenario 1. A video is presented of a supervisor berating and abusing an employee; 34 clicks later, it's time for the quiz.

*The best way for a supervisor to interact with an employee is:*

    A. *Call them profane names.*
    B. *Make fun of their personal appearance*
    C. *Threaten to beat them up*
    D. *Treat them with respect.*

No doubt, many of these ridiculous mandatories are required by third-party regulators. No doubt that many of the issues raised are important. No doubt, plaintiff attorneys will seek any and every opportunity to make an institution look bad if they can make some money off it. No doubt, the media may like to exploit the "lack of training" to embarrass a healthcare institution. But there needs to be some sanity and oversight. Each new mandatory becomes part of the regular work week for an administrator, but it must be done in the surgeon's free time.

# THE BREAKING OF THE SURGEONS

*Dear Leader Y,*

*I completed the four additional mandatory modules that were added this year. I believe this makes ~23 mandatory tutorials to complete every year, which is slotted in for well over 100 hours of time; of course, we can actually complete them much quicker. The four new modules are slated to take up to 2.5 hours each. They are ludicrous and mind-numbing and cannot reasonably be claimed to have any educational value.*

*I guess my real question is whether there is a process to review the necessity of all of these and whether the length/quizzes are appropriate. Of course, we live in the real world and many are requirements -- but we just seem to add a bunch every year. If completed as directed, it would probably take 2-3 weeks of full-time work to get through them, and I do not believe our billing targets are being reduced by 4-5% to facilitate compliance.*

*It is fine to have lectures and emails about burnout, but meaningful action would be far preferable.*

*Thanks for considering,*

*Neil*

Just a word or two about social media, as two words are more than enough to summarize what I know about these platforms. As a non-participant, I have heard many times how social media keeps you connected, keeps you in the loop and mitigates the fear of missing out (FOMO). Physicians have 24/7/365 electronic access to medical records, imaging studies and lab tests on multiple devices and to the healthcare team and patients around the clock by cell phone. Do you really think we need to be more electronically "connected?" I am blessed with JOMO (joy of missing out) and recommend it highly.

# Chapter 10: Academic Medical Centers

Academic medical centers (AMCs) have been the anchor and backbone of American medicine for decades. They are the epicenter for medical education, the developmental home for physicians-in-training, the birthplace of life-saving scientific discoveries and the providers of sophisticated, cutting-edge medical care. There is just so much history and achievement to be passed on to the next generations, who are often inspired and motivated by this spirit of discovery.

However, academic institutions have fallen into the moral trap of believing that this tradition of achievement in innovation, research and education immunizes them from remaining accountable, acting honorably and living up to their traditional, mission-based principles.

We seem to have convinced ourselves that pretty much anything we do can be justified by this elite standing as well as our historic role in caring for the underserved; we are the good guys. But AMCs are falling short in many, if not all of these areas. Many of us are too often focused on using the system to gain personal recognition and privilege. We have become lost along the way.

All sorts of actions and practices that just don't have moral face validity are enabled (or at least accepted) based on the fundamental belief of an AMC's intrinsic goodness. But how does an AMC justify refusing care to underserved populations? How do we justify incentivizing spending less time with patients than they need? What is the educational justification for essentially selling highest-level faculty appointments to attract high revenue-producing surgeons with no interest in teaching? Or rewarding excellent teachers with a pat on the back for their commitment and a cut in pay?

I was treated well as a faculty member in the AMC system (as I always was a high-volume surgeon), but there are so many examples of the fundamental disconnect between what we say and what we do.

As Robert De Niro said in *The Deer Hunter*, "This is this; this ain't something else. This is this!" And this is where the activity as a substitute for achievement smoke screen resurfaces.

We create this imaginary alternative reality with alternate facts where we are acting nobly and in accordance with our stated values and mission. A whole vocabulary of empty or misleading phrases is used to sanitize and effectively mischaracterize what is actually happening. Buying into this culture, using the C-suite lingo and messaging the faculty is a requirement for leadership in academics as well these days. Unfortunately, it is again the case of two parallel universes under the same roof.

This may be gratuitous, but I feel I need to make a few comments on background. First, I very much enjoyed and am appreciative of my career. Again, I was treated very fairly.

Second, I had a pretty traditional academic career with active participation in patient care, research, education and administration. I was well integrated into the system and can reasonably be held accountable for at least some share of the shortcomings, even though I was never shy about speaking truth to power. I never sought, applied for or wanted any higher level of authority in my institutions.

Lastly, as I like to wryly say, I was a philosophy major in college (actually true), so I can speak for hours on issues of little or no importance. Hopefully, you, the reader, will not emphatically agree. Apologies in advance to my teachers for any and all conceptual misrepresentations.

Empirical frameworks rely on weighing the impact of actions and seeking the greatest good. I have always found this very subjective and prone to distortion and moral ambiguity. Empiricism does not serve as a proper guide for the medical profession, at least as commonly employed.

In the present framework, the AMC promulgates the mantra that we are the good guys. We have lofty missions. Things that enhance our bottom line (even if they would strike the man from Mars as unseemly) should be considered good because we will have more money to support our missions -- and this is good.

This is how we can justify treating colleagues from other institutions unfairly. Or excuse the moral foibles of the high revenue-producing surgeon and make an example of the lesser one.

Or ride out of town a senior surgeon who has given selflessly to the institution but has become ill or less productive. Or indoctrinate medical record plagiarism as standard practice and incentivize profound level of service misrepresentations to charge the highest possible fee to patients that we can get away with. Or how we justify ignoring the needs of the un/underinsured patients. *No money, no mission.*

We cannot justify dubious actions on the basis of some greater good expectation -- that's a very slippery slope. In contrast, Kant and many rationalist or virtue-based writers focus not on what is good but on what is right.

Just do the right thing; actions should be guided by principles (or maxims). Treat people fairly and honestly. My take on Kant's message (with profound apologies to Kant and anyone who had me in one of their philosophy classes):

- Act as if the maxims of your action were to become, through your will, a universal law.

- Treat humanity not merely as a means to an end but as an end in itself.

- Whatever principle determines my action is the basis for morality.

- Goodwill is the only thing that is good without qualification.

## THE BREAKING OF THE SURGEONS

You are a surgeon walking into work at 5:00 a.m. You are deciding whether to stay on the pavement or take the short cut through the grass, which has just been seeded by the landscaping team. If you cut through the grass, you will get to your patients a bit earlier and have a little more time to spend with them -- this is good. No one else is there to see you and be influenced to take the shortcut either -- no harm, no foul.

But what if this were a universal law and everyone did it? Is it really true that cutting across the freshly seeded grass saves lives? It's just not the right thing to do, so don't do it. This is obviously a trivial example, but the point is that it is hard to know when four wrongs will really result in a right. It's easier, less confusing and more comfortable to act in a way that would make your mother proud. *Right is right; wrong is wrong.*

OK, down from the soap box. I am just a colorectal surgeon. According to a *Harvard Business Review* analysis, between 1975 and 2010, the number of physicians increased by ~50%, which was about the same as the U.S. population. The number of administrators grew by 3200%. With this, we saw the transition from the social compact of the healthcare profession to the transactional/conditional rules of a business.

Hospital CEO salaries grew from a mean of $1.6 million to $3.1 million from 2005-2015, a trend that only seems to have escalated in recent years. This is approximately 10 times more than the growth of physician salaries despite ~1/2 of the education. The ratio of doctors to other healthcare workers is now 1:16, down from 1:14 two decades ago. Of those 16 workers for every doctor, only six are involved in caring for patients -- nurses and home health workers, for example. The other 10 have purely administrative roles. So, there are 10 administrators for every physician -- that just can't be right.

Generally speaking, administrators are a pure cost center. As their numbers continue to grow exponentially, there are far more mouths to feed for those who actually deliver care. And typically, no one generates revenue like surgeons. Numerous administrative layers continue to be created as a substitute for understanding the nuances of healthcare delivery and to compensate for only vague notions of what may be important. With every new layer of bureaucracy, leadership is further insulated from reality and there are more folks to be thrown under the bus when needed.

It seems like every time there is a new concept in the magical lexicon of the C-suites, a senior VP position is created with yet another people pod to be crowded into the world of Zoom sessions, forwarding reply to all emails and agenda-free meetings. More departments and administrators seem to define the institution as being on the "cutting edge."

I recall when service lines were introduced in AMCs; it makes sense that physicians who work together in a multi-disciplinary manner to treat the same patients should be organized and care coordinated. I was named the co-Director of the Digestive Diseases Center at UVM. No one could really say what this meant, what was expected or what should be done. I also was the co-Director of the Digestive Diseases service line at UChicago. Again, there was no budget, no deliverables, no specific responsibility and no defined aim.

I asked senior leadership repeatedly to explain what they had in mind and we put together a set of strategic initiatives aimed at enhancing the teaching, research and clinical care missions; no response of any kind. We even had an administrator hired (a really good person with skills and initiative), but they were never provided any direction or charged with anything meaningful. They left. That's how it works -- the ones who want to get something done and have an impact leave; the ones who are happy to get paid handsomely and sit on Zooms all day, send emails and go to bogus committee meetings stay.

On a panel, I once heard Dr. Tom Fogarty define a committee as "a group of the unwilling, selected by the unable, to do the unnecessary."

Many of us work at academic medical centers because we want to participate in research. This is rapidly becoming an area where the activity-to-achievement ratio in administration has become the highest. History has shown the critical importance of participant protection in biomedical research. The Institutional Review Board

(IRB) has a very important role to play in ensuring ethical conduct and that proper safeguards are in place.

But somehow, over the years, the IRB process has morphed into wildly excessive paperwork and a "just say no" approach that stifles research. Generally, the overwrought caution, stonewalling and bureaucracy have little or no connection to patient protection and seem to have become encultured across the research enterprise.

Below is a typical response I received from an administrator when I had been waiting for a simple signature for almost a year for an IRB-approved project.

*Hi Dr. Hyman,*

*To provide an update on where things stand on our end, Y and I had completed the application that determines if a data request is for quality improvement or human subjects research, but shortly after, COVID erupted, and Y transitioned to her new role. In the interim, conversations with our internal data acquisition group and the Senior Project Manager occurred, though other departmental and sectional needs were prioritized over making significant progress on this project. We still need to connect with our internal University Research Administration and also determine if a Data Use Agreement needs to be in place in order to share this data.*

*Best,*

*X*

## THE BREAKING OF THE SURGEONS

*Dear Operations Manager X,*

*Read this again and again to try and figure out what you are saying.*

*Sounds like we dropped the ball and did not do what we said we would do — we just needed one signature.*

*Neil*

In a culture where activity is the coin of the realm and there is no need for any legitimate achievement, a huge chasm is also created between the administration and rank-and-file faculty. Those who derive from and report up to the luxury boxes just need to create the appearance of achievement to be able to play in the imaginary world of the fantasy football league. But researchers and other faculty have actual competitive grants to win and manuscripts to be accepted into high-impact, peer-review journals; the outcomes of that actual work is carefully measured, benchmarked and scrutinized.

Based on ignorance and a lack of familiarity, administrators must again rely on administrative PINOs and other physician leaders to bridge the gap between the two worlds. Unfortunately, many academic leaders have not stepped up in their zeal to show they belong in the luxury boxes and that they understand its language and culture.

With the massive infiltration and proliferation of business-trained leaders with no experience and limited understanding of the nuanced work of faculty, the rules and hierarchy of the business world have taken root and grown like weeds.

The practical impact is that administrators unload iterative work on physicians because administrators believe we work for them; the pyramid of priorities has inverted with the patient and medical education cast as the bottom feeders.

The role that the Dean and the medical school more generally play in the AMC has been severely curtailed in many healthcare settings.

Parenthetically, I would highlight that this is not the case at UChicago, which I view as reassuring and commendable. But in an ever-increasing number of medical schools, a series of "academic" figurehead leaders are chosen and given minimal authority, just so that the affiliated healthcare system can create the façade of an AMC.

There is often only low-level managerial power afforded to the physician leaders; the role in many "academic" centers could perhaps best be described as Accountant or even Puppet-in-Chief. There may only be a minimal expectation of a commitment to education or research, begging the question of what the definition of an AMC really is.

Medical schools have struggled mightily in this environment to fulfill their historic missions of research and education, because they are not usually the ones with the money and must walk around with their hand out to the healthcare system CEO for support.

What is the medical school supposed to do in this weak and compromised situation? It has been interesting to watch how medical schools try and preserve their relevance and mission, as their traditional values are often diametrically opposed to those in the C-suite.

To compensate for the absence of authentic promotion of humanism in medicine and doctor-patient relationships, a growing number of ceremonial awards are given instead.

Thankfully, speakers are becoming more diverse as DEI has received increased emphasis. But lecture series still usually feature a retired old White guy (like me) with an impressive white coat picture or suit (unlike me). He talks about the importance of spending time with patients, shared decision-making and justice issues surrounding healthcare access and disparities. These lectures can inspire but sound hollow in an era where professional ethics has become what we talk about and not what we do.

We get to pretend for 45 minutes before we go across the hall to our department meeting with senior leadership and the PowerPoint telling us we are spending too much time with patients and need to see more in less time. Even though there will be less access to patients as fewer folks will be able to receive care here (based on their relative contribution to margin), we will take even fewer transfers and OR access will be curtailed owing to the nursing shortage, we expect your case volumes to go up by 5%. The hamster wheel will be cranked a bit higher again this year anyway. *Run baby, run! Burn baby, burn*! As usual, there will be no operational accountability on the institutional side.

And by the way, your salaries will be frozen or cut in these "unprecedented times." After all, reimbursements are shrinking and costs are going up. We hope you do not review the institution's Form 990, as you will learn that we were able to increase the salaries of senior leaders by 15% yet again this year and reinforce their golden parachutes. There was no problem finding millions and millions of dollars to continue this precedent despite the "unprecedented times."

One of the best pieces I have read describing the present status of U.S. medical schools was written by noted cardiologist Dr. Milton Packer. It is excerpted below but I would recommend reading the entire article which appeared in *Med Page Today (November 2018- reprinted with permission).*

**Med Schools' Business Model Is Officially Dead**

**Milton Packer describes the slaughter of "academic" medicine**

*As the funding of healthcare expanded in the last 30 years -- particularly procedural revenues -- medical schools thought that they could recreate their business models by incentivizing their clinical faculty to grow their practices and referral base. But, doing so led to the creation and growth of massive health systems, giving administrators enormous financial power that did not depend on traditional academic structures or missions. Now, even at the most "academic" of medical schools, the clinical faculty are often paid directly by health systems; their employment and salaries depend on their ability to generate fees, not research papers, and their time is managed by healthcare and service line administrators rather than department chairs or division chiefs.*

*With health systems in charge, medical schools have become financially starved and have lost control of their faculty. The vestiges of the academic structures are still in place, meaning there are still deans, departmental and divisional leaders, people with educational titles, and students. But, unless they also have authority over the health system or service lines, the men and women in leadership positions are often only figureheads. They are relics of an obsolete structure which has no funding and little decision-making capacity. Unless you can direct the expenditures of state funds or philanthropic money, you serve at the pleasure of an administrator who often has little sympathy for any time spent related to research or teaching. Leadership positions at medical schools are increasingly filled by those whose primary qualification is demonstrated loyalty to the healthcare system rather than traditional "academic" credentials. All too often, these positions are filled by insiders who can be recruited with minimal resources and whose personal allegiances are well-established. If academic leaders pursue a parallel "academic mission," they do so at their own peril.*

*As a result, many deans at modern medical schools serve a ceremonial function. Like the English monarchy, they preside at events and say inspiring things to those in attendance, but they have no power. But, unlike the Queen of England, they typically have no money.*

*Now, "academic medicine" is dominated by a corporate model that cares little about any intellectual mission. Medical schools often propagate with little relationship to any academic faculty. The ceremonial and organizational vestiges of an interconnected bygone era are still evident, but they no longer mean what they used to.*

# Chapter 11:
# Quality

"Culture eats strategy for breakfast," observed Peter Drucker. Failure to appreciate the centrality of this adage to quality improvement has led the house of surgery into a stagnant rabbit hole. Surgeons understand and generally embrace societal expectations that we value our commitments to patients and society more broadly; that our status as a profession demands competence, self-regulation and altruism; and that we should be guided by a moral compass. This cannot be achieved by paperwork.

When I started at UVM, our Chair, Steve Shackford, was a staunch crusader for quality assessment and improvement in surgery. He made it clear that this was foundational for our identity as surgeons and made this the centerpiece of our culture, promotions and reappointment. This culture (complemented by rigorous peer review and authentic data collection) created a shared sense of mission, purpose and departmental pride.

For many years, I was Chief of General Surgery at UVM. I was always well aware of our key performance metrics and we reviewed our performance together on a regular basis. We used prospective data collection, tracked meaningful outcomes in real-time and used this as the primary basis for quality assessment and improvement.

## THE BREAKING OF THE SURGEONS

In my early career, I used to write a fair bit about quality improvement in surgery (what we would call "outcomes research" today), but I lost interest when the field seemed to decay and degenerate into an alphabet soup of organizations and form generation. Meaningful outcome measures were often too difficult to capture and the quality train left the station largely fueled by process measures…and without the overwhelming majority of surgeons on board.

The concept was promulgated that good process is a surrogate for good outcomes. If everyone only adopted the right processes of care, everything would turn out fine in the end. This had very limited face validity in actual practice and generally turned off the surgical community to the quality movement.

So, if a patient had surgery for rectal cancer and the tumor was left in place, an unnecessary colostomy created, both iliac arteries transected, both iliac veins injured, the ureters divided and the patient lost 30 units of blood, it was implied that the surgery should be considered "high quality" because a hair clipper was used instead of a razor for the preoperative shave.

Surgeons often were criticized for not being on board with quality improvement. No doubt that there are instances where this criticism can be reasonably leveled. But it was no surprise that the blossoming institutional gamesmanship that resulted from tracking superficial and/or clinically marginal process measures did not engage the surgical community. To most, our professional obligation was being "Dilbertized" by bureaucrats and silly initiatives were routinely rolled out and presented with sheepish apologies, arguing only that it was better than what some third party might impose.

Many of the committed surgeons who tried so hard on a national level to make things better and safer for patients are my friends. I have so much respect and empathy for the enormous challenges of herding cats and trying to improve quality across the broad spectrum of healthcare cultures, values and norms. Further, there have been a number of noteworthy achievements around the edges, such as the creation of quality collaboratives, informative databases and process standardizations.

However, the underlying strategy of quality by forms created a torturous bureaucracy, rampant inauthentic and ineffective initiatives and a "what will they do to us next" feeling among many surgeons.

Quality improvement came to mean more paperwork imposed by a largely sequestered group of clipboard nurses. Failure to achieve buy-in and inculcate a quality culture has been a lost opportunity. A commitment to continuous quality assessment and improvement has to come primarily from grassroots belief and commitment from the surgeons and cannot be imposed from the outside.

As Dr. Cliff Ko, a highly respected leader in the surgical quality space, observed in a 2022 *JAMA Surgery* commentary: *"Despite the volume of activity, evidence persists of preventable mortality and complications, inefficiencies, disparities, and unwarranted variability, suggesting that suboptimal care is a much less tractable problem than perhaps was anticipated at the dawn of the quality and safety movement. It is now clear that QI itself requires improvement."*

There have been notable successes and initiatives that do engage surgeons. Surgeon-initiated outcome collaboratives and prospective data collection, along with ongoing peer review, are key components in creating a quality culture. Although a bit out of favor these days, I still see a critical role for peer review conferences, probably for all the reasons I object to the top-down, forms-based approach to quality discussed previously.

There is no doubt that morbidity and mortality conferences often have been dominated by a select few whose views have become institutional doctrine based on intimidation rather than evidence. Although accountability remains a core attribute for a surgeon, there can be no justification for cruelty and shaming.

Around 10 years ago, I was asked to write one of the chapters for the American College of Surgeons quality manual about case review, along with two highly respected surgeon leaders. My views on quality and case review, in particular, are reflected below in this excerpted, largely unpublished section.

## THE BREAKING OF THE SURGEONS

*Case review is a time-honored, comfortable, and familiar forum for quality improvement that has been a cornerstone of surgical training and practice for decades. The idea that members of the healthcare team should meet periodically to review individual cases and seek to improve the end result of care was championed by Codman and others following the Flexner report.*

*Codman defined case review simply as "the common sense notion that every hospital should follow every patient that it treats...with a view of preventing similar failures in the future."*

*When approached properly, case review can meaningfully engage surgeons in the quality culture, as well as provide an excellent opportunity to lead and model professional behavior to colleagues and trainees.*

*Recent years have brought an intense focus on maximizing the value that Americans receive from our healthcare system. Value, in this context, means improving both the processes of care and patient outcomes while reducing costs.*

*On the quality side of this equation, there has been an extensive array of consortiums and agencies created to measure, assess and improve the efficiency and effectiveness of care of the surgical patient.*

*In this environment, case review has often been relegated to secondary status and not considered to have the precision, objectivity and global applicability of some of the newer initiatives. However, the quality improvement efforts and tools that are derived from these systemic efforts may confuse and intimidate surgeons, typically fail to engage them at the grassroots level, and may be viewed as sources of considerable angst.*

*Achieving consensus on a quality measure that can be applied in a uniform and meaningful way to all patients with a specific surgical disease can be exceedingly challenging.*

*Further, as Donabedian observed, "The most important outcome may be the least easy to measure, so easily measured but irrelevant outcomes are chosen."*

*The quality improvement principles that have been utilized so successfully in industry have been adapted to healthcare delivery and often serve as the template for these efforts. The Donabedian model of structure, process and outcomes has provided a useful framework for analysis and many papers have been written over the past two decades looking at how these attributes of our healthcare delivery system relate to the quality of care patients receive.*

*However, drawing correlations between structure, process and outcomes may have limited applicability when one tries to understand why an outcome has occurred in a particular patient treated by a specific surgeon at an individual hospital.*

## THE BREAKING OF THE SURGEONS

*There are so many potential confounding variables that the interpretation of relationships between care and outcome can seem to be a contrived and artificial endeavor.*

*In short, we often do not know what the actual driver of better outcomes is, so we may be challenged to design a rational quality improvement strategy applicable to every institution.*

*Certainly, looking at quality "from above" provides a panoramic view that can guide policymakers. While many of the quality improvement efforts at the organizational level (third party payers) have been focused on the process of care, only recently has an emphasis been placed on outcomes.*

*With the establishment of large patient registries populated with data gathered concurrently with care, such as the National Surgical Quality Improvement Project (NSQIP) and the Northern New England Study Group (NNE), not only the process of care but also the clinically meaningful outcomes of care, can be assessed and compared between institutions. This assessment can identify high-performing hospitals and determine best practices.*

*Occasionally, these large, national databases identify outliers that experience outcomes disparate from their normative peer group (either better than expected or worse than expected). Identifying these cases or trends can be quite useful in directing attention to problematic areas but should not be used as a proxy for local case review.*

*Case review provides for a local, grassroots look at the care provided by an individual practitioner to a patient in the specific and unique environment in which the care occurred. The patient-centered focus and the ability to review the course of care and associated circumstances along with peers working with similar resources provides a platform of relevance, truth and authenticity to assess process and outcome.*

*In addition to improving the quality of care, case review also fulfills the part of our social contract that provides physicians with autonomy in the affairs of medicine while self-regulating.*

*Case review, if performed well, achieves self-regulation. In this context, case review remains a critical component and perhaps the epicenter of meaningful quality improvement. Rather than relying on the speculative associations that are typically generated by database reviews, the surgical team can analyze exactly why a patient had an adverse outcome with a mind to prevent this from happening to future patients. This is the very essence of Codman's end result concept. While analyses of large administrative databases can demonstrate associations between certain practices or aspects of healthcare delivery and outcomes, they seldom provide a firm direction for quality improvement efforts at the granular level.*

*This is because data capture is generic and may not record all of the potentially confounding variables in a specific case, as there is much diversity and variability in the local environment where healthcare is delivered to a surgical patient.*

*If done properly, case review is a potent tool to promote team building and to create a true culture of quality that exemplifies professionalism.*

*In fact, there are few more meaningful expressions of a surgeon's professionalism than a regular and robust ongoing evaluation of individual surgeon and team performance that is accompanied by an ongoing vigorous effort to improve them.*

*This is the very essence of the social contract that surgeons have with their patients as professionals. Said another way, the relentless pursuit of promoting high quality patient care and safety is the bedrock of our professional identity and celebrates the sanctity of the doctor-patient relationship.*

*All surgeons are familiar with case reviews, as morbidity and mortality conferences have long been an integral part of surgical training and education. These conferences have been viewed as a "proclamation of accountability" and "the means by which a surgical apprentice is socialized into a surgeon."*

*Morbidity conferences provide surgeons with an opportunity to confront medical errors, openly discuss adverse events and learn from their mistakes and those of others.*

## THE BREAKING OF THE SURGEONS

*Surgeons play a key role in peer-reviewing cases of their colleagues to identify potential or real deficiencies in surgical care.*

*Despite the central role of case review in quality assessment and improvement, this modality cannot and does not stand alone. There must be mechanisms to define evidence-based best practices so that peer review is not dominated by adherence to local customs or the parochial beliefs of a particularly aggressive surgeon or surgeons.*

*Further, outcomes must be benchmarked against national norms so that specific areas can be highlighted for emphasis and particular scrutiny.*

*In this regard, NSQIP is an excellent complement to local case review. NSQIP can identify the procedures where there is the greatest opportunity for improvement and where local efforts are most likely to be fertile. But, it is through individual case review and assessment at the local level that specific systematic changes can best be designed and implemented. This must include a mechanism to ensure that the desired changes are occurring and that they are having the desired beneficial impact.*

*Case review must be conducted in a positive and constructive spirit, remembering that the goal is (as articulated by Codman almost a century ago) to determine the end result of treatment with the aim of benefiting future patients. Although surgeons and teams must be strictly accountable for patient outcomes, the focus must be on opportunities for improvement.*

*The determination of whether the care given to a specific patient was good, bad, optimal, or suboptimal should be based on the current knowledge supported by the best evidence and must be evaluated objectively.*

*When case review is viewed as an opportunity for "grandstanding" or to display hubris, the goals of the review and efforts at creating a culture of quality may be profoundly undermined.*

*As Hurwitt observed in 1965, "...it is not intended as a virtuoso concerto for a solo performer....but for the purpose of enlightenment that removes any unwarranted involvement of personalities."*

*A successful outcome of any case review is achieved by consensus and inclusivity and marked by the generation of a fair, logical and feasible plan for process improvement.*

*Importantly, there must be a mechanism to ensure implementation of the action plan, which typically includes designating the person or persons responsible for each step in the plan along with a timeline. There must also be metrics developed to define success and a plan made to assess whether the desired quality improvement has occurred.*

*There are several factors that improve the effectiveness of case review. First, there must be commitment to participate by all disciplines involved in the care of the surgical patient. This starts with committed leadership.*

*Second, the process of review must be explicitly defined. Operational definitions of specific adverse events and complications should be provided to all participating departments in advance of implementing the case review process. Doing so early can eliminate concerns of bias for or against any individual. Having an explicitly defined process with precisely defined adverse events will add clarity and facilitate the process.*

*Third, reviews must be concise. Elaborate processes with multiple steps should be eliminated, keeping in mind that all members of the team have time constraints.*

*Email communication is not inherently a work product. As legendary college basketball coach John Wooden stated, "never mistake activity for achievement."*

*Lastly, and perhaps most importantly, the institutional leadership must commit to providing the resources and the backbone to assure that actual quality improvement, rather than the appearance of quality improvement, occurs.*

*Although consensus should typically be sought, there are occasions in which consensus cannot be achieved. In such instances, the leader must decide and do so objectively and with integrity. Leaders must remember that not all adverse outcomes can be attributed strictly to a systems problem; undisciplined, unprofessional or unsafe practices require principled action.*

*When repetitive problems with a single provider are identified, a formal peer review process should be implemented. Similarly, when outcomes from a surgical procedure fall below national benchmarks (NSQIP observed/expected ratio), a multi-disciplinary review is indicated.*

*The modern morbidity and mortality (M&M) conference should have the ability to unite the new technology of large database outcomes reporting, such as the ACS-NSQIP program, with the time-honored tradition of individual practitioner case review and open discussion by peers and members of the multi-disciplinary team.*

*A benefit of database reporting is providing more accurate and complete outcomes with up to a full 30-day window of follow-up. This is important since traditional systems have multiple flaws, which can lead to underreporting of complications, primarily those that occur after hospital discharge.*

*The importance of surgical leadership and an institutional commitment to quality cannot be overstated. The Chief of Surgery (or designee) must assure fidelity to the case review process. An energized but fair peer-review process and a clear expectation of accountability is critical for the establishment of a quality culture.*

*Participation in quality efforts and peer review should be required as a condition for receiving operative privileges. The institutional Board of Trustees must assure that the administrative leadership provides the resources necessary to support these efforts fully.*

*Statutory peer review protection from discovery of the results of peer review is pivotal in ensuring complete disclosure of information obtained during the review of adverse events. The goal of case review must be to provide the unrestricted and free flow of information and opinions necessary to make patient care as safe and effective as possible, not to provide a resource for plaintiff's attorneys wishing to promote malpractice litigation.*

*Although we fully concur with a constructive and systems-based approach to quality improvement, we also believe that case review (e.g., morbidity conference) loses much of its performance improvement and cultural value if individual responsibility and accountability are not highlighted, as well as the dynamics of systems and team function.*

*As Prasad observed, "Concern for hubris may not be in vogue the way 'checklist' and 'systems failures' are, and yet, like other truths of human nature, it plays an important role within medicine." He added, "To omit from medical practice and reflection those countless cases where misfortune evokes humility, responsibility, remorse and even agony is surely to strip the conference of the title, 'golden hour.' To discuss error without these sentiments is ephemeral and doomed. The M and M conference is about more than patient outcomes and cannot be understood simply in the language of 'systems.'"*

# Chapter 12:
# The Data Dump

Although there are exceptionally talented surgeons and a rich tradition of surgical advances to be proud of at UChicago, authentic quality improvement efforts were generally met with the same administrative indifference described earlier.

It seemed like the institutional attitude was, "We know we are really good, so let's just fill out the forms and get it over with."

It is often said that if you torture the data, it will confess to anything. Selective use of data, especially out of context, is a potent bedrock of the activity vs. achievement smokescreen. So much data is available from so many sources and databases that one can quickly put together cleverly "curated" PowerPoint presentations to make it look like some sort of earnest assessment has occurred.

When I was in New England, we had put together both a statewide and then a regional colorectal quality collaborative. The key impact was on the creation of an authentic quality culture, collaboration, learning from each other and defining best practices.

Having initiated these efforts, I am well aware of the broad-based, institutional resistance commonly encountered by my surgical colleagues. Administrators don't see the value of these collaborations for their institution and lawyers worry about the risk of data collection.

Because we had values-based leadership in Steve Shackford at UVM, we really had very little or no pushback. But many of our colleagues were tormented mercilessly by their "academic medical center" when trying to join.

I really saw the difference between institutions where surgical leadership embraces a quality culture versus trying to contend with it in the least painful manner.

I had hoped to help cultivate the same culture at UChicago, but I confess that the indifference and passive resistance wore me out. We shifted focus to more broad-based, national initiatives.

*Dear Senior Leaders X and Y,*

*I really do need some help with this. As I alluded to several months ago, the issues with our "quality" folks is beyond poisonous. To review, we participate in a number of quality collaboratives this one is the "AA" collaborative. As leader X knows, we got caught up in an email extravaganza that lasted over a year with changing requests every time we met in person until we finally got things moving.*

*It was time in May for our next data dump - you can see below that our colorectal champion was involved in 43 emails (yes, I counted them) simply to have data forwarded. I have done a lot of database quality work over my career and I know that essentially none of this is necessary. Thankfully, I know the principal investigators well and they have been willing to put up with our unique inability to get pretty much anything done without a hassle of epic proportions.*

*In addition to not having my junior colleague abused like this, I am very concerned because this will be a major focus of our newest faculty's research activity and there are several, major national efforts underway that will really provide her some amazing opportunities to be a leader in colorectal quality initiatives. She will have no chance in this unsupportive environment. I would very much welcome your suggestion for someone senior who might work with us to change the culture and related processes so my young guys can have a fair opportunity to be successful.*

*We have been dancing around with this since August of 2018: unanswered emails, misinformation, broken promises, false assurances and on and on.*

*Do not know why this is necessary.*

*Thanks,*

*Neil*

Meaningful quality improvement requires a true partnership between surgeons and the institution. Sometimes, there is low-lying fruit and there can be quick wins so that unsafe or suboptimal practice can be remediated. Examples include antibiotic stewardship, checklists for standardized processes and hand washing.

Unfortunately, it is usually more difficult to institute policies and procedures that apply across the board to the complex and nuanced challenges encountered in patient care.

Two competing narratives are often generated about quality initiatives. Sometimes, surgeons complain about being forced to practice "cookbook medicine." But we really do need to acknowledge that there are situations where there is no good reason for variability in practice and it should be eliminated whenever appropriate. Standardization of routine processes generally makes surgery safer.

But requiring and rewarding standardization when there is a legitimate need for individualizing care undermines surgeon buy-in. No one appreciates being pushed to add the "official" approved prophylactic antibiotics for patients with resistant organisms, where the required antibiotics may be ineffective. No one is engaged by the inevitable gaming that often occurs when the institution focuses on improving an artifactual metric.

For example, it had been suggested that normothermia decreases wound infections after surgery, an association that has subsequently been shown to be suspect.

A typical institutional response would be to avoid measuring the temperature in the first hour postoperatively since patients often arrive in the recovery area cold and take a while to warm up. The clipboard quality team is then congratulated by senior leadership for the "improvement." What surgeon would be engaged by this?

The newly created quality alliances tried very hard to thread the needle between having meaningful process measures and watering them down to allow for reasonable and appropriate variability. But the focus on process created a bureaucracy built around clipboard nurses that seemed to turn quality into a game, equated quality with form completion in the minds of surgeons and generally provided for little if any improvement in the quality of care.

Anytime a new "quality" initiative was announced, eyes in the room would start rolling and the "what are they going to do to us next" looks would ensue. What a shame.

As Donebedian and others have noted, outcomes are the truest measure of quality. This concept has strong support in the surgical community. But to paraphrase, meaningful outcomes are hard to measure, so easily measured but irrelevant outcomes are chosen instead. Of course, this is a poor way to engage the surgical community.

The Leapfrog Group was founded in the 2000s largely by healthcare purchasers to "improve the quality and safety of American health care." Letter grades are assigned to hospitals based on various measures of patient safety, such as the use of computerized order entry and e-prescribing. A few surgery-related metrics, such as hospital and surgeon volume are included, but the assigned grades cannot reasonably be considered a comprehensive guide to surgical safety.

Further, the relationship between performance of Leapfrog measures on outcomes is, at very best, dubious and has been refuted in multiple studies.

If a patient comes in for a vein stripping and loses their leg because the femoral artery was mistaken for the saphenous vein, I doubt the patient and their family would be satisfied and feel comforted because postoperative pain medicine was e-prescribed. It's just not reasonable for surgeons to feel engaged by Leapfrog as the backbone for institutional quality.

At UChicago, our performance year after year on Leapfrog was consistently outstanding. There is a legitimate reason to be proud of this and highlighting this data was the cornerstone and workhorse for our messaging on surgical quality. We were also members of ACS-NSQIP, which provided far more meaningful data that benchmarked our outcomes against our peers. These reports engage surgical teams because they are generally regarded as authentic. This data was very hard to come by and rarely shared.

# THE BREAKING OF THE SURGEONS

*Dear Leader X,*

*I know I have raised this issue a number of times, but I think it is really important that the Chiefs be aware of how we are doing relative to our peers on quality metrics. I understand that we preferentially show the Leapfrog data each time there is a quality report, and it's nice we do well; I am sure we can agree that risk-adjusted mortality, readmissions, and major postoperative complications are more authentic metrics of quality than written policies for handwashing, bilirubin measurements in babies, ICU staffing, use of e-prescribing, etc.*

*Thanks again for considering,*

*Neil*

For some operations, the outcomes of interest generally can be agreed upon. If you have heart surgery, you don't want to die, you don't want to have a stroke and you don't want to have heart failure. But is death/stroke/heart failure really a good way to discern who is a high quality hernia surgeon? Wouldn't you want to know the incidence of hernia recurrence and nerve injury instead? But how would you go about getting that data? What would be the gold standard for determining "recurrence" and who would make this impartial assessment?

Or who should a patient see for a hemorrhoidectomy? Again, does a low rate of death, stroke and heart failure characterize a high-quality hemorrhoid surgeon? How would we measure and capture recurrence, continence and hygiene issues post-op? Codman did it far better over 100 years ago. He kept index cards for all his patients and kept track of his results (including what we would now call patient reported outcomes) -- my kind of guy. Indeed, culture eats strategy for breakfast.

Well-meaning quality programs have been developed at a national level for quality improvement for a number of surgical diseases. Again, I would make the argument that they often miss the mark by focusing on process measures with arbitrary compliance targets.

For example, in the case of rectal cancer, key consensus elements of quality care are multi-disciplinary input/review, high-quality MRI, high-quality surgery and high-quality pathologic review. How best to achieve this really depends on local factors and logistics, including resource availability and the population served.

No surgeon celebrates being pushed to order a CT of the chest, abdomen and pelvis and an MRI of the pelvis in an elderly patient with a palpably unresectable low rectal cancer and advanced dementia. No one should feel good or be complacent about having this patient's daughter take three days off of work and exposing her mother to unnecessary and even invasive tests just to comply with externally imposed, arbitrarily derived metrics. It may not be a big problem in Chicago, but it was a major issue in rural Vermont.

One of the most striking and glaring omissions in national quality efforts is the failure to appreciate the inherent variability in healthcare environments and patient values across the U.S.

When I practiced in Vermont, patients may have had to travel several hours each way to get specialty care. "Failure to test" was not because the surgeon did not know what test to order, as in the elderly rectal cancer patient with advanced dementia above and clearly expressed advanced directives. A digital exam was often all that was needed to direct quality, compassionate and responsive care.

Patients who live in rural and/or noncoastal areas do so for a reason and their values should be respected. They often wish to have care close to home, accepting in some circumstances that fewer resources may be available.

For example, foregoing radiation and several hours of daily travel for 5-6 weeks in the setting of a node-negative rectal cancer could be a very appropriate choice since radiation in this setting slightly improves local control but not overall survival.

When elderly rural patients developed diseases or a complication that was likely to be terminal, many times they did not wish to be transferred hundreds of miles away from home to have a heroic attempt at "rescue," especially if the most optimistic outcome was to spend a few months in a nursing home before passing.

"Failure to rescue" sometimes meant respecting the care preferences and values of a well-informed patient. And "rescue" seems a poor choice of descriptors for the outcome in patients who were transferred far away from their families, only to survive for another month or two in a debilitated state after undergoing many invasive procedures. It is important not to over-generalize, but the fact is that many patients in rural settings have very different values and life philosophies.

Chicago was a very different situation as most everyone lived in reasonable proximity to advanced specialty care. The barriers to access were largely cultural and systems-based; patients in the same city had very different access and were treated very differently based on their insurance status, demographics and where they lived. This created all kinds of challenges for patients, communities and the surgeons as well.

## Chapter 13:
# DEI

I became president of the American Society of Colon and Rectal Surgeons (ASCRS) in the aftermath of the George Floyd tragedy. To define my preexisting biases, I guess I am somewhat of a fiscal conservative and social liberal. I am generally skeptical that money will fix everything and I wish government and institutions more broadly were more respectful and thoughtful with how they spend other people's money.

But I believe that people should let other people live their lives as they see fit and allow them to be their authentic selves. Clearly, neither side of the political spectrum seems to be on board with this.

From the right, various people's lifestyles and identities are mocked and denigrated. But from the left, there is also mocking and disrespect of many people's values and perhaps a more subtle way of excluding people.

With that said, the concept of creating a more diverse and inclusive society was always something I thought about and valued. So, it was quite comfortable for me to elevate a group of ASCRS members who had been meeting independently for several years to become a standing DEI Committee and support the implementation of several initiatives.

I genuinely appreciated the opportunity to hear their ideas and engage in cordial, forthright and productive discussions on a fundamental issue I believe in deeply.

I did not want us to settle for one of the cosmetic or performative efforts that were in abundance. There was a lot of talk about "creating a safe place" for dialogue, but it seemed everyone knew that there was really only a single set of perspectives and statements that were expected.

This felt like a lost opportunity. I was enthused about supporting sincere and realistic plans, like improving equity in colorectal cancer screening and treatment. In a message to the membership, I said:

*"As the American Society of Colon and Rectal Surgeons, this should be in our wheelhouse and something we should be well-positioned to address."*

But I was not interested in signing on to letters espousing particular political positions that defined correct thought and instructed people how to think; that's being exclusive, not inclusive:

*"I would also like to highlight the need for respectful dialogue, acknowledging that all of us, by our very nature, have implicit bias. We have all had different experiences based on gender, race, socioeconomic status, sexual orientation, region of the country, rural vs. urban, academic vs. private practice, etc. and we need to be willing to acknowledge our experience and seek understanding."*

# THE BREAKING OF THE SURGEONS

As an old White guy, I got a lot of feedback after my initial message to the membership that others promoting a focus on DEI probably would not. For example:

*Re: A Message from ASCRS President on Diversity and Inclusion*

*Dear Neil,*

*With respect to your position and accomplishment, I really don't feel that the ASCRS has ever had a problem with "diversity and inclusion." I have always felt that our society promotes and is made up of one of the most diverse and eclectic groups of surgeons you can imagine. Well-represented by both genders, all races, and multiple nationalities. We all get along. It is one of the aspects of colorectal surgery that I think adds to its interest.*

*I really don't think we need a task force and all of the other things you mentioned to address the issue of Diversity and Inclusion. I see this only as an institutionalized effort of our society to be politically correct and to try to keep pace with the ridiculous craziness running through our country currently.*

*Thanks for considering my viewpoint.*

*Sincerely,*

*J*

## THE BREAKING OF THE SURGEONS

I got a number of similar, respectful emails from colleagues who I knew to be fundamentally good, earnest and honorable people. I appreciated the opportunity for constructive dialogue; this seemed so much more productive than forced indoctrination. I was also surprised how often DEI was considered to be a zero-sum game.

To elevate one group, we need to diminish another group. Or to consider the viewpoint of one group of people necessarily undermines the perspective of another group. It's a mistake to restrict expression to a single, officially-sanctioned viewpoint -- other than being committed to diversity, equity and inclusion as a core value.

*Dear J,*

*I really appreciate your writing and understand your point of view. I guess the bottom line is that a lot of our members do not feel included…and have written to let me know. There is a group that has been meeting for three years (the current task force) as they believe they have not had the same access to leadership/committee positions and speaking opportunities. There are lots of other folks who have written that they feel the leadership is very inbred and want to feel they have an opportunity to be part of the "in crowd". My experience has certainly been like yours, but of course, I want all of our members to feel the way you and I do.*

*I have met by Zoom with the committee a couple of times…they are very reasonable and sincere. Whether it's race, gender, rural vs urban, or academic vs private practice, I want folks to feel like they are one of us and enjoy the camaraderie we have.*

*I understand how you feel, but I would respectfully ask that you keep your mind open for a bit longer and see how this all works out. Please do keep sending me your thoughts and keep me on my toes/on point.*

*Hope all well,*

*Neil*

There are so many lessons to be learned and complex issues that we need to work through together as a society. There is too often a rush to judgment without the facts, which can have tragic and devastating consequences. Facts matter, and implicit bias is not restricted to one group of people; we all have it. We all draw conclusions and make generalizations based on our lived or perceived experiences. Sometimes, these lead us astray.

There is rampant fear in academic medical centers that someone will say the "wrong" thing and that what they say or do will be misinterpreted. Or, in rare cases, they will be falsely accused of something. All of these can be career-threatening.

As a result, most people just don't express their opinions and keep their views (and questions) to themselves unless they are sure they are among like-minded colleagues, or they just parrot the official talking points and required viewpoints of the thought police to keep safe.

I recall chatting with one of my highly respected senior colleagues several years ago while waiting for an elevator in the hospital. I was going up and he was going down. The elevator door opened and there was a young woman alone in the elevator heading down. He did not get in and hit the down button again once the door closed. I assumed this was because he wanted to continue our conversation. He then told me that he does not get into an elevator when there is a woman alone and no other witnesses as he fears a false accusation.

Now, I think this is extreme and know of no one else who feels this way -- but it is out there. Consider the rush to judgment two decades ago with the Duke University lacrosse players whose lives were devastated by false accusations and the vitriolic response of their classmates, Duke faculty, local authorities and community groups who jumped on the bandwagon before knowing the facts. We all have unconscious biases and can make mistakes generalizing from previous perceptions and experiences. There is a need to be mindful of our tendency to prejudge.

The response of academic medical centers and universities more broadly has been very disappointing. In my limited experience, when it comes to issues impacting race, gender or other hot-button issues, there is a calculated rush to judgment to "get ahead" of things before the actual facts are known. The calculation is made strictly based on what narrative is most politically expedient, how best to message the situation and the surest way to avoid controversy/upsetting the wrong people. The facts become almost irrelevant.

If the person accused makes the institution a lot of money, the issues will tend to get swept under the rug if at all possible. If the person is considered expendable, they will get thrown under the bus so leaders can use the situation to send the "right message."

To paraphrase Kant, treating a person as a means to an end without respecting their inherent worth is a grave moral failing. Our universities have largely taken up the position of leading from the rear and often seem to stand for nothing in particular. They typically try and timidly navigate the waters to avoid any and all controversy.

Again, I am a true believer in the academic medical center and especially the critical importance of universities as the unshakable home of free speech, earnest and respectful exchange of ideas and principled action. They are often anything but that now and it is very sad. No one learns, we do not challenge our own assumptions and we become divided and plagued by lowest common denominator viewpoints.

These sorts of pressures are not new. When I was in college, speakers with left-wing viewpoints often were prevented from speaking because of their use/views on marijuana or other mind-altering substances, their critiques of the Vietnam War, our system of government or other mainstream institutions. It was important to me (and an expectation as a student) that I would be exposed to and learn from as many views as possible. Any attack on free speech and freedom of expression was predictably met by student protest and resistance. So many of these counter-culture warriors were my heroes.

Perhaps it is generational, but I appreciate the opportunity to hear those with points of view out of the mainstream. It feels like a privilege to have my thoughts and assumptions challenged and an important reason why one chooses to work at a university.

I see protest (non-violent) as inherently healthy and a right to be cherished. But to see so many speakers and perspectives barred from campus is a real tragedy for an open society. It pains me to see students preventing people who they do not agree with from speaking, hunkering down in their hermetically sealed echo chambers and being coddled when they are at risk of having their views challenged.

If you feel that being exposed to other points of view is too upsetting for you, don't go to a liberal arts institution. To watch so many university leaders stand for little else other than their own viability, functionally denigrate free speech as a core value and hide fecklessly behind the ivory tower, is a real shame.

## THE BREAKING OF THE SURGEONS

The University of Chicago has a rich and cherished history of promoting free speech on campus. As William Rainey Harper, its first president said, "There is not an institution of learning in the country in which freedom of teaching is more absolutely untrammeled than in the University of Chicago."

This core value of the University always made me proud and has been reiterated many times throughout its history. The most recent iteration with which I am familiar was advanced in 2014 and is excerpted below:

*"In a word, the University's fundamental commitment is to the principle that debate or deliberation may not be suppressed because the ideas put forth are thought by some or even by most members of the University community to be offensive, unwise, immoral, or wrong-headed. It is for the individual members of the University community, not for the University as an institution, to make those judgments for themselves and to act on those judgments not by seeking to suppress speech but by openly and vigorously contesting the ideas that they oppose. Indeed, fostering the ability of members of the University community to engage in such debate and deliberation in an effective and responsible manner is an essential part of the University's educational mission.*

*Of course, the ideas of different members of the University community will often and quite naturally conflict. But, it is not the proper role of the University to attempt to shield individuals from ideas and opinions they find unwelcome, disagreeable, or even deeply offensive. Although the University greatly values civility, and although all members of the University community share in the responsibility for maintaining a climate of mutual respect, concerns about civility and mutual respect can never be used as a justification for closing off discussion of ideas, however offensive or disagreeable those ideas may be to some members of our community."*

Amen!

One area that I had respectful disagreement with was the separation of institutional DEI from the broader obligation to promote a more just, diverse and inclusive society; not just making our faculty and leadership more diverse but addressing healthcare disparities with genuine intent. I do not believe these two issues can be readily separated. At UCM, we did a really good job with the first but were relatively feckless on the second.

It was unsettling to accept policies that undermined our ability to care for underserved patients. Whether it was dysfunctional systems that impaired access, institutional decisions that largely excluded the underserved or the 16-hour waits to be seen in our Emergency Department, it was difficult to reconcile the expressed commitment to DEI with the lived healthcare experience we provided for our vulnerable neighbors.

# THE BREAKING OF THE SURGEONS

*Dear Leader Y,*

*I appreciate you and everything you do.*

*Really don't think I am alone in this re my perspective. As an institution, we routinely deny care to established patients who are really suffering (almost always patients of color), even when continuity of care is critical to outcomes. We don't even provide support or guidance as to where they can receive the needed care elsewhere, leave it to trainees to tell the patients and have a totally unaccountable and non-transparent "appeals" mechanism. There is no opportunity to explain the situation -- just a bare bones form.*

*In this context, the 12 paragraph email stump speeches about our values from senior leaders on every imaginable occasion really ring hollow. These issues are not easy but a sincere and meaningful effort to address instead of a smokescreen of empty rhetoric would be greatly appreciated.*

*Thanks*

*Neil*

When we could get sticky, foundational issues to the highest levels of the organization, the gaslighting would start. An egregious case, policy or procedure would be cast as a "one off" exception, even when everyone knew (or should have known) that it was a standard bill of fare. The lack of ownership, accountability and responsibility we exhibited in caring for our South side neighbors was very disappointing and sometimes overtly distressing -- talk is cheap and emails do not cure cancer.

*Dear Nurse X,*

*I am sorry to say that she was denied surgery here and the residents were told to find her somewhere else to be taken care of-no help or guidance was provided for them regarding how to operationalize. This was morally distressing and hurtful for them.*

*This patient got sick again and I appealed once again on her subsequent admission. We have been waiting for weeks for authorization to colonoscope her so she can have surgery. Our residents (and I) have spoken with her several times and tried to reassure her we would work on her behalf to try and cut through the red tape.*

*Unreal to get yet another unsigned form letter of denial and we are being forced to neglect her once again. I am sure (or at least hopeful) this is unintended. Not sure where to forward this as no one willing to be accountable for these decisions and the refusal letter is unsigned per this unaccountable protocol. I guess we have no choice but to send into cyberspace again and hope.*

*Thanks,*

*Neil*

From one of my junior colleagues:

# THE BREAKING OF THE SURGEONS

*Hello –*

*I get that everyone is helping on this case. And understand it is not one person's fault.*

*But I really don't understand how this patient can be getting treatment at U of C for the last year (including oncology, radiation oncology) and 7 business days before a surgery that was scheduled a month prior, we are notified that we don't have insurance approval and the surgery might need to be cancelled. Now, we are asking him days before a major colon and bladder resection to find a new primary care physician to get a referral?*

*I am not sure what to do, but I will reiterate that he has been off of chemo since we booked surgery and cancelling at this point could cause significant harm.*

*I have cc'd my chief Dr Hyman and his oncologist to see if they have any ideas.*

It is easy to make speeches and throw stink bombs from the gallery when you are not the one responsible for these decisions. An institution does not exist in a healthcare delivery vacuum; there are limitations as to what can be achieved in the setting of broad-based systemic problems and the legitimate institutional need for fiscal responsibility and financial viability. But it was the relentless use of spin, sanitizing euphemisms and the seeming unwillingness to confront complex issues earnestly that was so troubling. What do we really mean as an institution on Chicago's South side when we say we need to improve our "case mix?"

On the other hand, there was genuine interest in creating a diverse and inclusive faculty at UCM. In our department, diversity of faculty and an academic focus on DEI were pretty effectively addressed. But it seemed somehow disingenuous that almost every other lecture at Surgery Grand Rounds in recent years was DEI-related. Perhaps this is unfair and unduly skeptical, but much of it rang hollow in light of the failings with respect to our local community. Many of the talks were excellent and thought-provoking, but others were repetitive and weak. Although well intended for sure, it always seemed patronizing when faculty felt compelled to reflexively give over-the-top congratulations and kudos to any talk on DEI. Again, this often suggested/messaged an officially sanctioned and required viewpoint.

*Dear Leader Y,*

*No doubt the residents and junior faculty take notice when we work hard to be diverse and inclusive in our faculty recruitments……and when our senior faculty line up to make congratulatory remarks at the end of every DEI talk- this is great. But they also notice when certain patient populations get treated as second class citizens (second class often being a generous term); no*

OR access, no bed access for transfers, limited access to the assigned faculty, and no access to timely care in our ED.

I understand that healthcare equity is complex and a separate issue (to some extent). But it is related to a DEI culture and it matters; we need to earn the trust of our community one patient/one family one encounter at a time. They don't come to Surgery Grand Rounds.

Appreciate,

Neil

Dear Leader X,

We have made major strides in creating a diverse faculty with an inclusive environment. But, it is critically important to understand the impact of interactions with our community in promoting diversity, equity and inclusion.

Our house staff, nurses, faculty and staff are regularly exposed to our failings week in and week out, often causing moral distress and promoting burnout when we fall short. Instead of an anonymous, unaccountable system where requests for care continuity are reviewed in a "cone of silence," there should be a system we can be proud of that represents an earnest effort to provide a just solution.

*Certainly, caring for the underinsured is a complex issue. The faculty may not agree with a decision, but at least they were given the opportunity to advocate for their patient and know that the needs of the patient were known and considered.*

*I just wanted to highlight a few things:*

*I was on call for colorectal for 10 straight days during the school holiday week. Of the three patients admitted with diverticulitis in need of an elective operation after cool down, none had insurance U of C accepts, so the residents had to call around to find a colorectal surgeon who would provide the necessary follow-up and care. I think we know the "demographics" of these patients.*

*I do NOT think this is an easy issue, but I am really bothered by the chronic misinformation that this applies to 2-3% of the patients -- this has no face validity. This issue was raised by another surgeon in the ambulatory directors meeting as many are having an awful time with it; senior leader Y explained that the reason was "we do not want to disrupt the South side ecosystem"…will leave it at that.*

*Thanks*

*Neil*

Despite the foregoing, surgeons and nurses would typically continue to fight for their patients, no matter how many barriers were thrown in front of them and how much apparent indifference they encountered.

As pointed out in an earlier chapter, our healthcare system has remained viable based on the commitment and professionalism of nurses and physicians. But it cannot last forever as the personal toll to do the right thing drives burnout and eventually the risk of a mass exodus.

I stand fairly accused of a gratuitous shout-out, but I was always so proud of my team and wanted them to know it:

*Dear Guys,*

*Every patient admitted to UCM with a colorectal issue deserves the highest level of care we can offer. The fact is that we build bridges and earn trust with our marginalized community one patient and one family at a time, by showing respect, caring and advocacy……not just by writing papers about them, "messaging" the importance of DEI on certain holidays or giving each other awards.*

*Sorry for the melodrama, but it really is an enormous source of pride for me that our residents know we care about them and all of our patients. Although you are all obviously extraordinarily talented surgeons, it is perhaps your character and commitment I appreciate most.*

*Thank you*

*Neil*

Speaking freely, encouraging diverse perspectives and listening respectfully are essential bedrocks of higher education. Paradoxically, it is some university DEI offices where the dangers of creating a monolithic perspective have become most apparent; this approach can end up restricting diverse views if it mandates adherence to a "state-sponsored" framework of allowable thought. It would be wrongheaded and unfair to paint DEI initiatives with this broad brush. Indeed, I found our DEI folks and the University of Chicago in general to be very open, intellectually honest and willing listeners.

The University of Vermont was a whole different story and highlights the risks to intellectual freedom and even basic fairness when one perspective dominates and adherence to doctrine is strictly enforced by empowered thought police.

In my almost 25 years there, I encountered issues with students and our surgery residents interfacing with this system that truly boggled the mind and seemed beyond rational belief. Just speaking the truth was taboo if it was inconvenient for the officially sanctioned viewpoints. Issues here are sensitive and often difficult. Over my career, many important and badly needed societal changes have occurred, calling out sexual assault and many kinds of inappropriate behavior.

No doubt, balancing the rights of a victim with the rights of the accused can be very challenging, although I personally find it difficult not to believe the overwhelming majority of reports by victims. But understanding the impact of overzealous policies and broad overreach on the university community is critical, especially if policies are generated in an inbred anti-intellectual echo chamber.

For example, one can reasonably legislate that those in a superior position should not date those who report to them. But where does that leave surgery residents? Should we ban a PGY-3 from dating a PGY-2? Should we be surprised that highly intelligent people with similar goals and interests working in the same small town or city may enjoy each other's company? What does this say about the perhaps 1/3 of surgeons/physicians married to other surgeons/physicians or the 1/2 married to partners who work in healthcare? Didn't they once have a first date? Were they really all at the same PGY level? Should we require all of their marriages to be annulled to stay on faculty?

In light of their rigid adherence to doctrine, perceived moral superiority and unwillingness to consider other reasonable perspectives without the threat of retribution, I used to think of the Affirmative Action and Equal Opportunity Department (AAEO) as North Korea comes to UVM.

Instead of promoting diversity, equal opportunity and freedom of thought, I found AAEO to be a place where a particular bias was nurtured and systematically indoctrinated and where bigotry found comfort, community, support and encouragement. There were changes occurring there in my last years and I hope they now allow rational and respectful deliberation instead of weaponizing dogma and stigmatizing language to make an example of these young people.

It's not just UVM where only some viewpoints on DEI are functionally permitted. I was invited to visit the Brigham, one of the most storied and important academic institutions in the world.

When I met with the surgery residents, many were upset by the recent removal of the portraits of surgical legends from the historic auditorium where they had their educational activities, strictly because they were White men.

Of course, not all spoke and expect there were some nuanced views. But the ones who did (men and women) expressed their sense of betrayal and disappointment; they were very proud of the Brigham's history and the landmark achievements in advancing surgical care for patients around the world. They clearly found meaning in being part of these traditions.

As a former resident John Kass noted in his blog:

*"My plastic surgery alma mater, the Brigham and Women's Hospital, removed all 31 of the gold-framed portraits of its surgical chiefs from the surgical amphitheater where Surgical Rounds and Morbidity and Mortality Conferences were held.*

## THE BREAKING OF THE SURGEONS

*They were portraits of men such as Dr. Harvey Cushing, who founded neurosurgery, Dr. Dwight Harkin who inserted the first heart valve and developed the concept of the ICU, Dr. Francis Moore whose 'Metabolic Care of the Surgical Patient' saved patients from surgical shock, and my own chief, Nobel Laureate Dr. Joe Murray, who performed the first successful kidney transplants.*

*Were they racists? Absolutely not!*

*But some Harvard medical students complained they were 'uncomfortable' because the portraits were of only White Men!*

*And just like that, Voila! Dr. Elizabeth Nabel, the past president of Brigham Health, summarily removed all the portraits to more private spots. They were segregated so as not to upset the new women and men of science. At least it was just portraits and statues that were canceled.*

*Dr. Jeffrey Flier, former dean of Harvard medical school, said removing the portraits did nothing to promote diversity and wrote an op-ed condemning the cancellation of these medical giants.*

*Contradicting Dr. Nabel, who said no one complained, Dr Flier said many faculty were afraid to dissent, adding, 'More than anything else, the explicit fear of speaking out against this by faculty at all levels drove me to write this piece. I felt that I had to do this and that others more vulnerable to false criticism might then speak their minds.'"*

DEI and respect for others is not a zero-sum game. There is no need to demonize and stigmatize some to make room for the voices of others. It's not necessary to take away the basic rights of one group to enable the rights of another group. It's not necessary to hate or scorn one group of people to value another group. That is not diversity, it's not equity and it's not inclusion.

Everyone's voice should be welcome as long as it is not hateful. Our universities and academic medical centers should be the vanguard of inclusion and free speech. Disappointingly, they often fall short in promoting vibrant, authentic and impactful DEI agendas.

We need to focus on meaningful action instead of self-serving and disingenuous performances. How can we acknowledge and add the unrecognized accomplishments of various underrepresented groups without feeling compelled to bury the inspirational humanitarian achievements of others as required compensation? How can we make things easier for those whose needs are not being adequately addressed?

For example, what specific policies can we institute to support early-career women who are choosing to start families? It's nice that there are now lactation rooms, but what about adding more faculty/staff to enable more flexibility during pregnancy and early childhood years instead of more administrators?

How can you not be heartbroken by the 2021 *JAMA Surgery* paper by Erika Rangel et al. showing how awful pregnancy outcomes are for young women in surgery? Most of them continued their grueling work schedule consisting of greater than 60-hour work weeks and frequent night calls, often right up until the day of delivery. Two hundred and ninety of the surgeons surveyed (42%) lost a pregnancy, more than twice the rate of the general population.

Compared with non-surgeon partners of male surgeons, female surgeons were almost twice as likely to have major pregnancy complications: 48.3 % of them….48.3%! It's a disgrace and shameful that we let this happen to our young colleagues -- through ignorance and systemic neglect. We should have looked out for them.

## Chapter 14: Reflections

I believe things will eventually get better for surgeons, but I expect they will continue to get worse for a while longer. I don't think anyone seriously believes our present healthcare delivery system is sustainable, but it is the nature of leaders to hold on to their positions and protect the status quo. Patient care is largely sustained by the professionalism of doctors, nurses and other healthcare providers. Healthcare administrators continue to place additional burdens on care providers, making the practice of medicine and surgery increasingly more difficult and less satisfying.

This relentlessly increasing burden cannot be sustained and things may need to implode before they get fixed. A real tipping point occurred during the COVID crisis. We have reached that point where there are now so many administrative folks crowded and sequestered into the luxury boxes that the magical thinking of the fantasy football league has become the *de facto* operational reality.

There is a critical mass of highly secluded people calling the shots who have no idea what is going on. And as Machiavelli observed, "the great majority of mankind are satisfied with appearances as though they were reality."

I have never met anyone in the luxury box who means anyone any harm. I have met several whose arrogance blinded them to reality and others who were all about maintaining their position and cared little about the impact of institutional inertia on patients, faculty and care providers. It is really disappointing when these are physicians because they know or should know better. Respect for the social compact, having the values of the medical profession and a moral compass should be prerequisites for the luxury boxes, not disqualifiers.

Moral injury derived from being powerless to operationalize professional values leads to burnout. The ever-increasing barrage of garbage that rains down on the playing field destroys institutional cohesiveness and job satisfaction. Leaders cannot sit in the luxury boxes designing plays based on make-believe; there are real struggles in the trenches and providers actually have to block and tackle. Virtue should not be virtual.

Surgeons need role models and iconic leaders, not just managers. Business skills make sense and are probably an asset in the complex environment of healthcare. But the surgeon-in-chief cannot just be a timid, self-serving manager. I had so many incredible role models that were critical to my professional development, sense of belonging and pride in being a surgeon.

Role models and earnest mentorship have certainly not disappeared, but there is just not enough of it. The burnout rate in surgery is approaching 80% in some settings, leading to highly skilled and committed surgeons leaving the field and straining many others to and beyond their limits.

Surgeons need to be given control of their local environment, as they know it best and need to be valued and treated with respect. The priority pyramid needs to be inverted with patients moved to the top, providers in the middle and management on the bottom, instead of the business model where patients languish on the lowest level of the food chain.

We need to return to the days when leadership welcomed the partnership, insights and observations of the "working" physicians and wanted to understand how best to serve their community instead of how to make a buck. Again, I think back to the days when the hospital president at UVM ate lunch in the cafeteria with the staff and wanted to know what was going on -- and what we needed to make sick patients better. We were part of "us." It's amazing what the truth, a sense of mission and legitimate inclusion does for camaraderie and morale.

The administrative response cannot just be a free cup of coffee on National Doctors' Day or access to yoga mats. Iterative work needs to be sharply curtailed, processes streamlined and meetings with no agenda and no deliverables eliminated.

As a workplace culture, folks need to be expected to solve problems and not just be part of bogus departments that forward their work to the physicians. People need to be retrained and discouraged from the routine use of reply to all emails. I do not need to be informed that someone in accounting is bringing Tostitos to Melvin's retirement lunch, that we are changing trash can vendors next month, or that all went well with the monthly generator check.

Surgeon leaders need to stand up, push back and advocate for patients and their teams instead of trying to ingratiate themselves to the luxury box gatekeepers. We especially need to be mindful of the vulnerability of residents and young surgeons who rely on us to ensure a supportive and healthy workplace.

The qualifying bar to a surgical career seems to get raised every year and the accomplishments of these kids are off the charts. They are the best and brightest of their generation and deserve to be treated as such. We have let them down. It is hard for surgical newbies to effectively fend for themselves against the administrative machine at a time when they are trying to establish their professional identities and learn the unwritten rules.

They have typically been overachievers their whole lives, at the very top of their class and every comparative ranking. They often have no experience with failing. If we let them be treated like a hamster on a wheel, they will just run themselves to death to meet or exceed targets that may be unreasonable. Administrators don't have to live like this; if there is more work, they just hire more staff. Have we ever had to consider duty hour restrictions in the C-suite?

Surgeons need to reestablish themselves as institutional messengers rather than accept strictly being messaged. We should all remember that it was not a long time ago when surgeons were treated as "we" and not as "them" by their institution. Why is it standard workflow that surgeons come back in from home after a 12-hour work day or sit in the surgeon's lounge all night long, waiting for the five minutes needed to drain an abscess in a terrified young man with severe pain? Because it was deemed "cost-effective" to close a room during daytime hours? Or more likely, the needs of the patient and surgeon were of little or no importance to OR administration, as there was no budgetary impact of failing to get the case done during the day?

Surgeons are responsibility takers in an environment where others often shun responsibility and look to pass the buck. They are decision-makers in an environment where decisiveness is often lacking, yet at a premium. Perhaps above all else, they are all about accountability for their outcomes, decisions and efficiency among other things. These attributes should be cherished instead of taken for granted.

In the end, an administrator will never understand that there is no off switch in the world of surgery, especially in the electronic era. When people used to ask me what I did for a living, I always thought I should answer that "I worry." I worried every day of my career about anastomoses leaking, that my patients would recover from surgery without incident or that their cancer or IBD would recur. Surgical care (at least good patient care) is fundamentally a personalized, mom-and-pop operation.

Teams are invaluable and there are many underutilized opportunities to rely on colleagues and teammates. But responsibility and accountability cannot be outsourced. I have never liked the "doc du jour" strategy that we so often see in other specialties. Tests get repeated, key details are lost and the wheel is constantly reinvented. Thankfully, we have started to see some pushback and an understanding that this approach is way more expensive, less effective and a real source of patient frustration/dissatisfaction.

Senior leaders often think about surgeons in generic organizational staffing terms. We need four cardiac surgeons, five colorectal surgeons, six vascular surgeons, three breast surgeons, etc. They don't seem to acknowledge that referring physicians and patients most often wish to see a specific surgeon and not a surgeon du jour -- that is until the leader or one of their family or friends need a surgeon. Somehow, there was no longer the need for a 16 hour wait in the ED to be seen, getting through to the clinic or finding OR time.

Patients don't want to talk to "a nurse." They want to talk to a nurse knowledgeable about and familiar with their condition, who has the ear of their surgeon. They don't seem to realize that patient problems in their "staffing models" do not get resolved and just recirculate endlessly in cyberspace.

One of the surgical leaders I admire most recently wrote me, "I am encouraged by the younger, up-and-coming physicians, including surgeons who clearly will drive changes in the system. They will simply not tolerate some of the 'stupid things' expected of them."

The English poet Edward Young said, "Affliction is the good man's shining time." I hope that those of us further along in our careers will have the back of these talented and committed men and women and help them shine. They deserve it, our patients deserve it, and academic medicine desperately needs it.

## About the Author

Dr. Hyman retired as Professor of Surgery and Chief of Colon and Rectal Surgery at the University of Chicago School of Medicine in 2023 and is Professor of Surgery Emeritus at the University of Vermont College of Medicine. He has authored over 250 peer-reviewed original articles and textbook chapters.

He served on many regional and national committees and is a member of many national organizations and societies. He has been President of the Vermont Chapter of the American College of Surgeons and chaired the American College of Surgeons Advisory Council for Colon and Rectal Surgery, the Council for Advisory Council Chairs, the Crohn's and Colitis Foundation Surgery Research Network and served as a Director of the American Board of Colon and Rectal Surgery. He is a past president of the American Society of Colon and Rectal Surgeons (ASCRS) and serves as Associate Editor of the *Annals of Surgery* and the *Journal of Gastrointestinal Surgery*.

Dr. Hyman is the recipient of many teaching awards, including Clinical Teacher of the Year, University of Vermont, College of Medicine (1993-94, 1994-95 and 1997-98). He received the Jerome S. Abrams Teaching Award in 1992-93, 1993-94 and 1997-98, the Howe Outstanding Surgery Faculty Award 2000-2001, 2004-2005, 2010-2011 and the Humanism in Medicine Award, University of

Vermont College of Medicine in 2001-02. He was chosen Teacher of the Year by the Chief Surgical Residents in 1991, 2007, 2009, and 2014 at UVM and at the University of Chicago, where he received the Robert Baker Award for Excellence in Teaching in 2015, 2016, and 2017.

Dr. Hyman received the 2022-2024 Mentor Award from the ASCRS Research Foundation and was designated as a Master Clinician at the Bucksbaum Institute for Clinical Excellence at the University of Chicago. He was selected as Physician of the Year by the Vermont State Medical Society in 2011 and received the Distinguished Academic Achievement Award from the Alumni Association of the University of Vermont College of Medicine in 2014.

He received his B.A. from the University of Pennsylvania in 1980 and his M.D. from the University of Vermont College of Medicine in 1984. He completed his surgical residency at the Mount Sinai Medical Center in New York and his colon and rectal fellowship at the Cleveland Clinic Foundation in Cleveland, Ohio.

www.ingramcontent.com/pod-product-compliance
Lightning Source LLC
LaVergne TN
LVHW051036070526
838201LV00009B/215